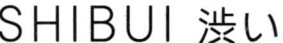

SHIBUI 渋い

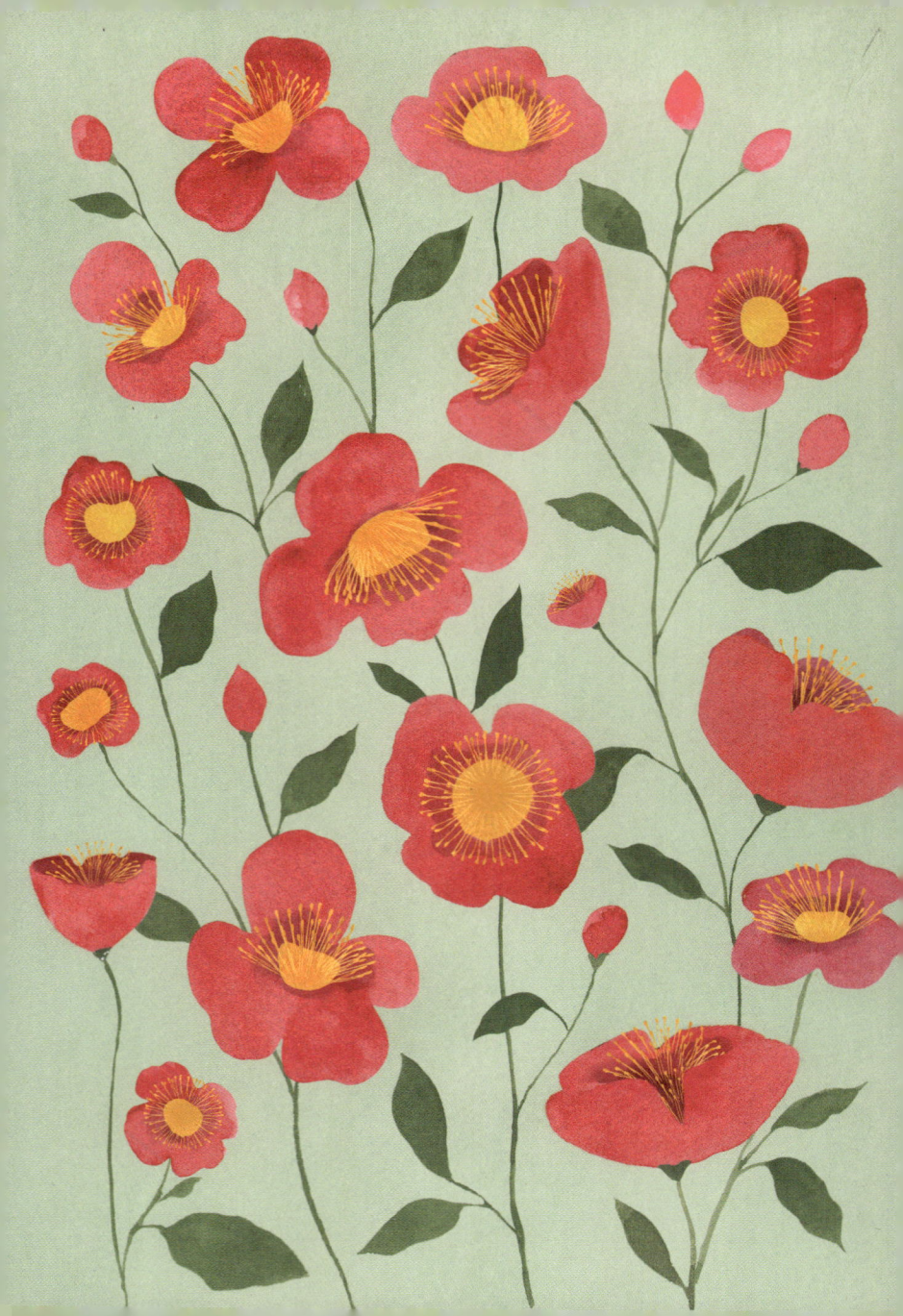

渋い

SHIBUI

THE JAPANESE ART OF FINDING BEAUTY IN AGING

SANAE ISHIDA

SASQUATCH BOOKS | SEATTLE

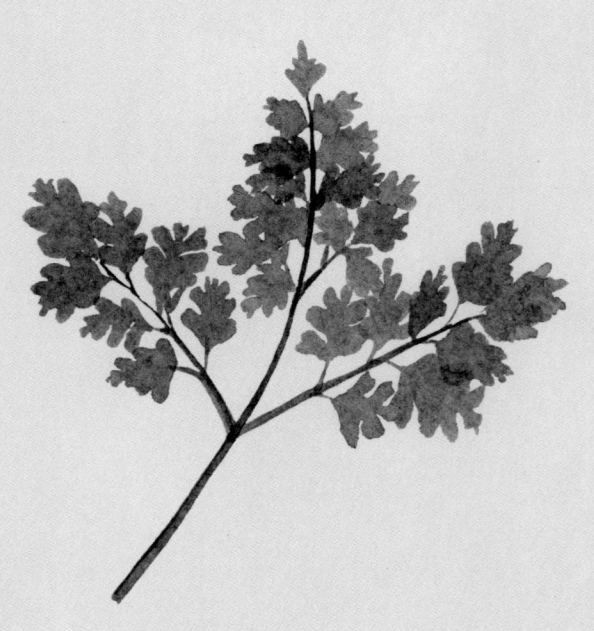

TO HANNAH, WITH SO
MUCH GRATITUDE

TABLE OF CONTENTS

ix *Introduction*

1 BI / BEAUTY

3 On Beauty

7 Imperfect Beauty

13 How Long Until a Beautiful Place?

17 Winsome Wisdom

19 First (In) Sight

21 Wrinkle Reading

27 KENKŌ / HEALTH

29 On Vitality

31 The Joy of Menopause

35 The Benefits of Restraint

39 Put Your Hands Together

41 Nourishing the Whole Self

43 How Are You?

45 MOKUTEKI / PURPOSE

47 On Purpose

49 The Loop

51 From Nothing to Something

53 Retirement: Redefining Purpose in Later Years

55 Tantanto and the Middle Way

59 White Envy and Urayamashii

61 Shigoto Hard, Play Hard

65 TOMI / WEALTH

67 On Measuring Wealth

69 A Very, Very Rich Life

73 Keeping Up with the Joneses and Shibuis

77 Supporting Roles

81 Bountiful Leftovers

83 Wanting What I Have

89 TSUNAGARI / CONNECTION

91 On Connecting

93 Wizened and Intertwined

97 Lost

99 Universal Interconnectedness: Serendipity

103 Even the Yakuza Respect the Elderly

105 The Loneliness Dis-Ease

109 Carless in Seattle

113 OWARI / THE ENDING

115 On Dying

117 The White Mustard Seed

119 Ichigo Ichie (and a Story About Tigers and Strawberries)

123 The Aftermath (Afterlife) and Quirming

125 The Crows

129 Kireizuki

133 *Conclusion*

137 *Glossary of Japanese Terms*

145 *Acknowledgments*

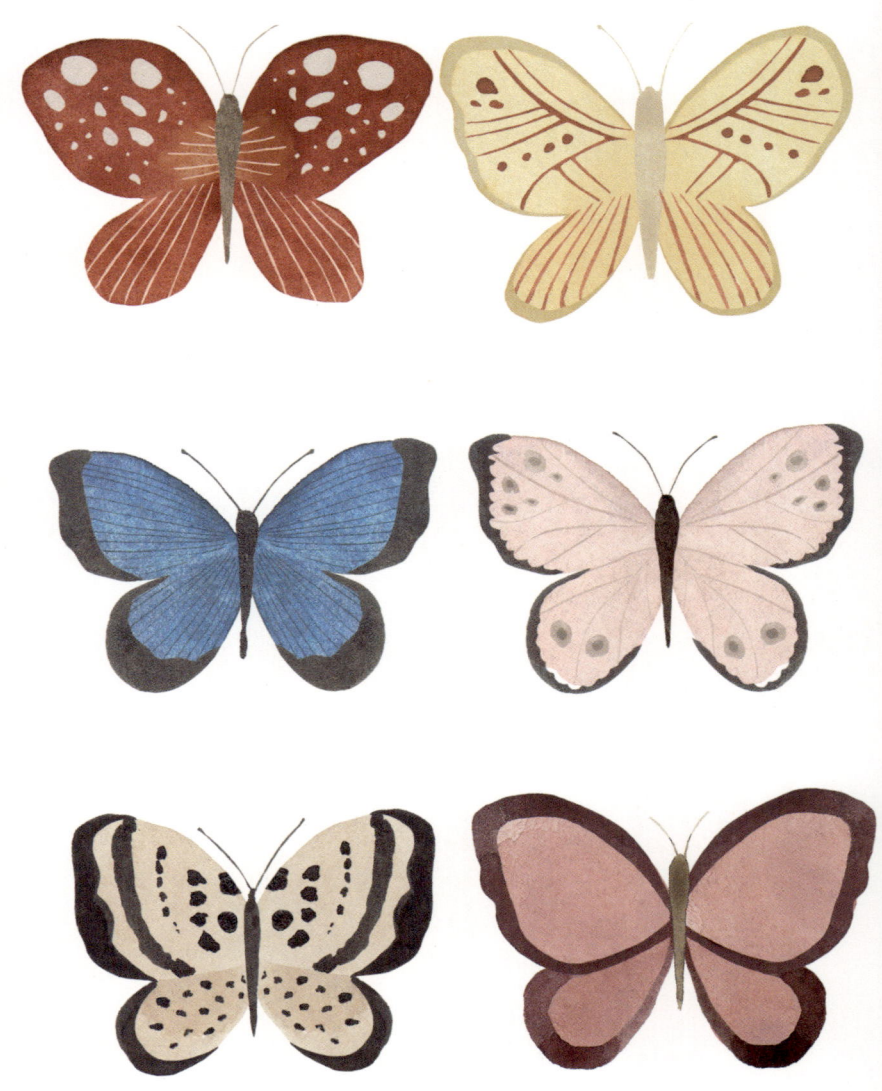

INTRODUCTION

I THINK A LOT ABOUT aging and death. Perhaps it's my Japanese-American upbringing; my Tokyo-born mother constantly talked about dying from the time I could grasp language. It wasn't as morbid as it sounds, although she regularly tossed out comments like, "I wonder how long I have to live," or "I want to make sure I do *x*, *y*, and *z* before I die." Death and mortality are a part of our daily conversations, simple facts to be acknowledged.

Growing up in Los Angeles, California, I learned that the typical American regards the topic of death as quite the opposite. Here in the United States, I found that the *D* word was not to be mentioned, and any sign of advancing age felt taboo, especially in the neighborhood near Hollywood where I grew up. "I'm already saving up for Botox," a grad school friend once told me. He was in his early twenties.

There are certainly aspects of contemporary Asian culture that promote obsessing over the maintenance of a youthful appearance for as long as possible too (K-beauty, anyone?). Alarmingly, I have heard that because of the omnipresent youth-worshipping messages on social media, preteens have been caught shoplifting anti-aging creams from Sephora! Urban myth or not, it's not surprising; aging is treated as a serious problem.

I started dyeing my hair to cover the increasingly prominent gray strands when I turned forty, a little over ten years ago now. Noticing my graying hair felt uncomfortable. At some point I had accepted that the fading color equaled old, which held a bad connotation. But why? When I closely observed the silvery gray roots, they looked lovely—sparkly and festive, like natural jewelry. Yet I covered the silver with a dark brown hue for six years until the high maintenance became too much. My pocketbook suffered, my pillowcases and towels got stained, and the hours at the salon added up and felt wasteful. On my forty-sixth birthday, I decided to stop coloring my hair. Now at fifty-four, my hair is about half-gray, and I love it.

This journey with my hair mirrors the essence of what I've come to understand as *shibui* aging—learning to appreciate the natural changes that come with time; finding beauty in authenticity rather than artificial preservation. We are *meant* to age.

The Japanese adjective shibui is a nuanced term with many definitions but no exact English analogue. The noun form is *shibumi* or *shibusa*, and it describes a distinctly astringent and slightly bitter aftertaste commonly associated with biting into an unripe persimmon. As the persimmon ripens and matures, the bitterness lessens. It may not disappear entirely, but it's no longer the dominant factor. The concept connects acrid unripeness with youth and sweetness and pleasure with maturity.

Shibui also conjures an image of a subtly sophisticated and mature object or person. Dr. Soetsu Yanagi, a Japanese philosopher, potter, and founder of the *mingei* folk art movement, popularized the term in the 1930s. He outlined seven elements of shibusa: simplicity, implicitness, naturalness, modesty, everydayness, imperfection, and silence. In essence Dr. Yanagi viewed the concept as the encapsulation of mindfulness.

The word carries a here-and-now awareness on the one hand and a well-worn yet timeless quality on the other—both of which are anchored with a profound appreciation for life. Shibui often applies to tangible things such as people, handmade crafts, art, garments, and architecture, but it is also used to describe the ineffable quality of an atmosphere or lifestyle.

I remember my mom using it synonymously with "cool," as in James Dean cool or Audrey Hepburn charming. The word very much encompasses the sort of aging I want to undergo: mindful, simple, beautiful, and all-embracing. Shibui is a wholly accepting word. It is a paradoxical, non-dualistic, and multi-layered concept that doesn't exist in English.

What does it mean to embrace a shibui attitude as we experience the progression of time? I have some thoughts that are guided by the ancient Eastern practices and teachings I absorbed through my Japanese heritage, balanced by the Western attitudes I've learned as a woman born and raised in the United States. The Japanese culture treats elders with immense respect and reverence, which is not something I see as often here in the United States. But I also see value in the individualistic, expansive, and experimental characteristics often prioritized in the West. In this book I take a Western experimental attitude and apply it to a distinctly Japanese concept.

Throughout the book, we'll explore shibui aging through various lenses: beauty, health, purpose, wealth, connection, and ultimately, our relationship with mortality itself. Each chapter offers both cultural insights and approaches to welcoming this stage of life. Rather than fighting against time's passage, we'll discover how to appreciate the upsides—the deepening wisdom, the liberation from others' expectations, and the subtle beauty refined by maturity.

I hope you enjoy this journey with me to find joy, wisdom, celebration—and yes, beauty—in aging.

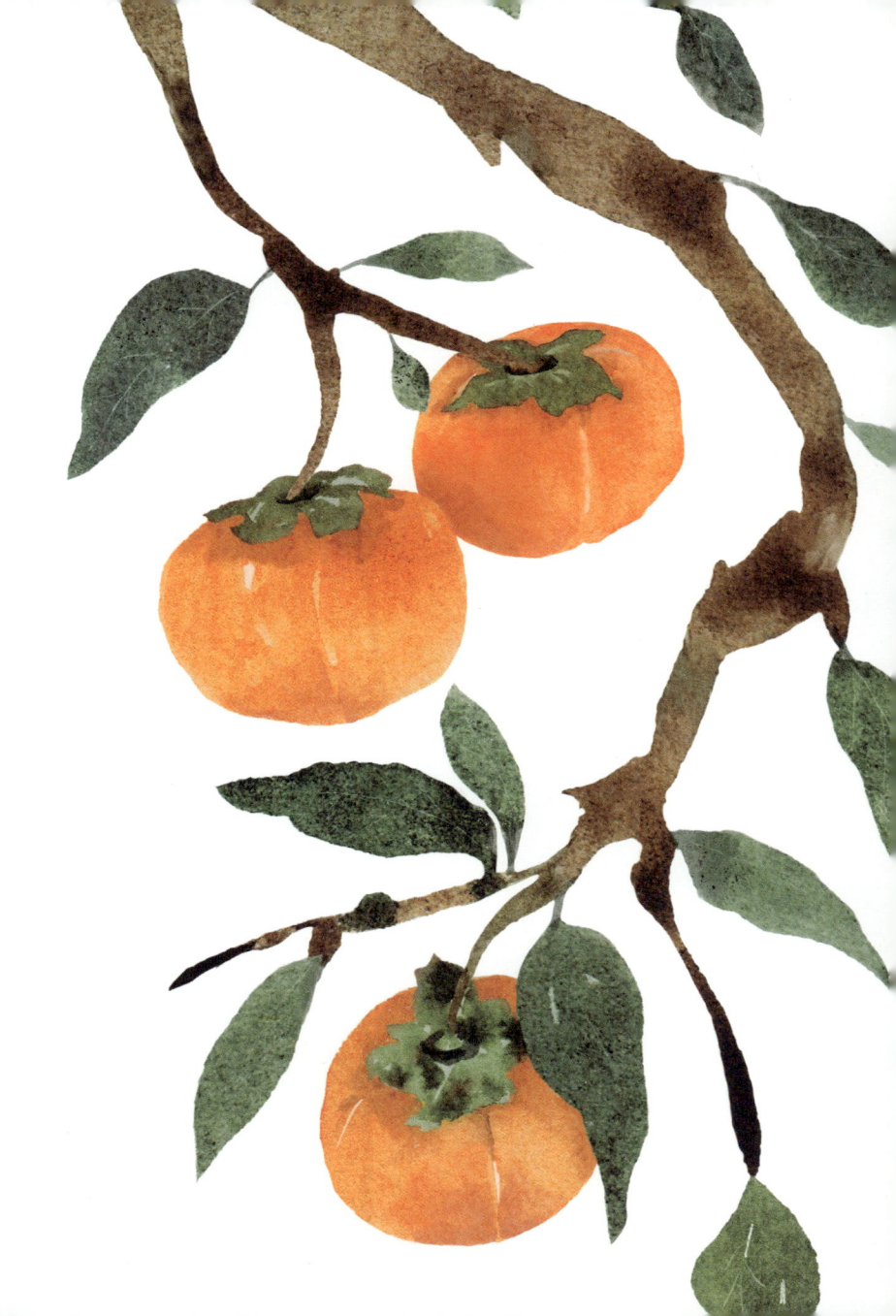

Shibui (shih-BOO-ee) . . . refers to a kind of beauty that only time can reveal . . .

HOWARD RHEINGOLD
They Have a Word for It: A Lighthearted Lexicon of Untranslatable Words

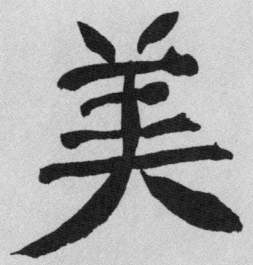

Bi

BEAUTY

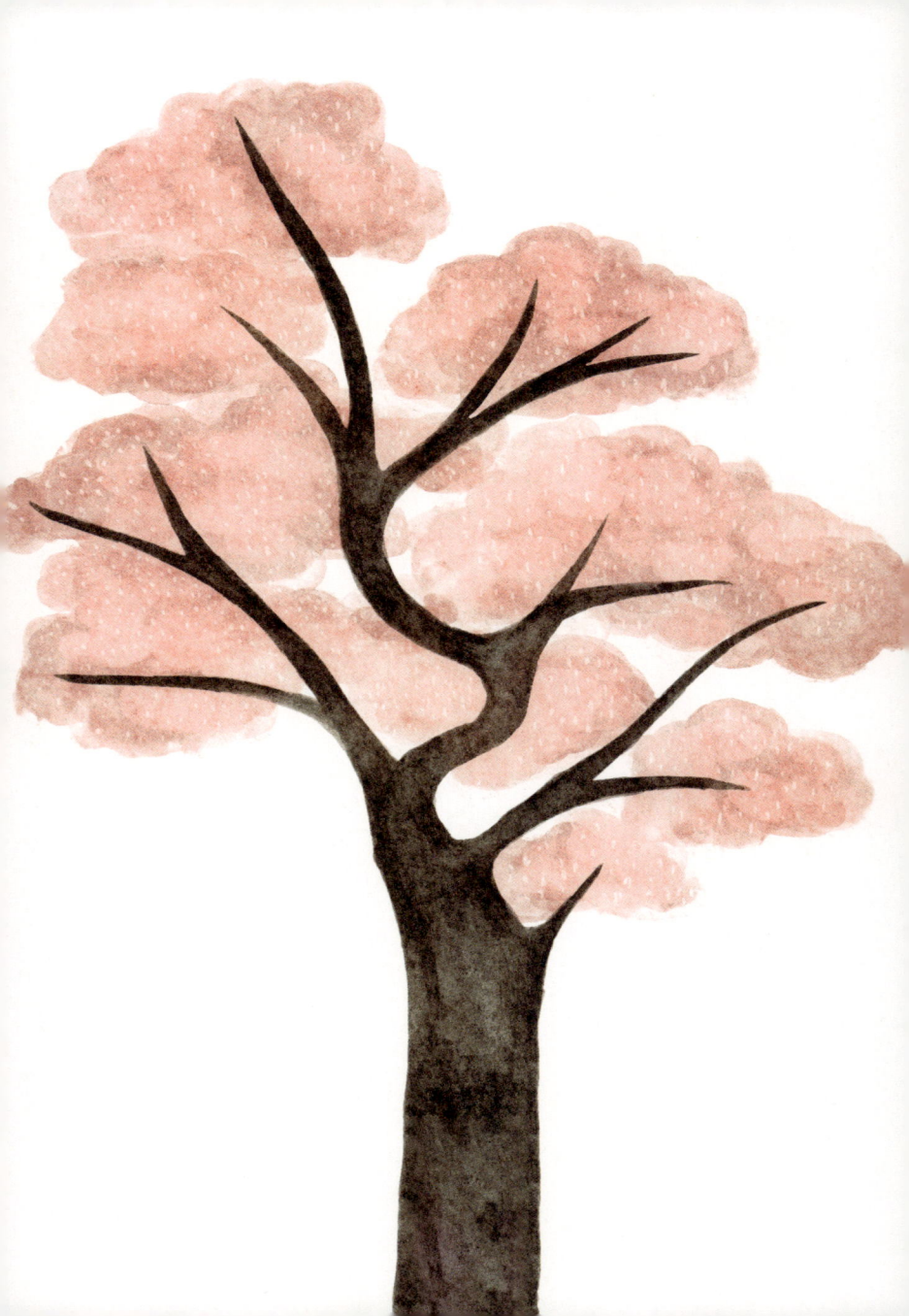

ON BEAUTY

GROWING UP IN LOS ANGELES, I was surrounded by
the pervasive idea that beauty is external, overlaid upon
our hidden interior selves, something to be consumed
from the material world—a skin-deep, one-dimensional
view. I internalized an unspoken assumption that beauty
is static and standardized, forever young.

Shibui, a concept from my Japanese heritage, offers a
different perspective. While Western ideals often seek to
overlay beauty upon us, shibui suggests that true beauty
emerges from within, revealed and augmented by the
passage of time.

Consider how a tree gains character with each passing
year or how a well-loved leather bag softens and pati-
nates. This is the essence of shibui: a harmony between
the inner and outer self that deepens with age.

Just as the skin holds its shape in a balance of internal
and external forces, shibui beauty arises from a similar
interplay. It's not just about appearance but how our inner
landscape—our experiences, wisdom, and character—
shapes our outer expression.

In my twenties, I worked at a non-profit theater
company housed in the Center for African and African

American Culture. My bosses—both performing artists and a former couple turned business partners—were rapidly approaching conventional retirement age. He showed up for meetings in snazzy, bold-hued zoot suits and tap-danced while playing the saxophone for his shows; she was a renowned actress and teacher of theater, guiding incarcerated women in telling their stories onstage. I couldn't help but notice how ageless and graceful they seemed despite the evidence of time marking their faces and bodies. Their combined experiences orchestrated elegant, heart-soaring performances that could only be described as shibui.

Shibui beauty transcends the material world. It's in the way a grandparent's eyes crinkle with joy, the unselfconscious full-throated laughter erupting from women of "a certain age," the gentle hands of a lifelong gardener marked by sun and soil.

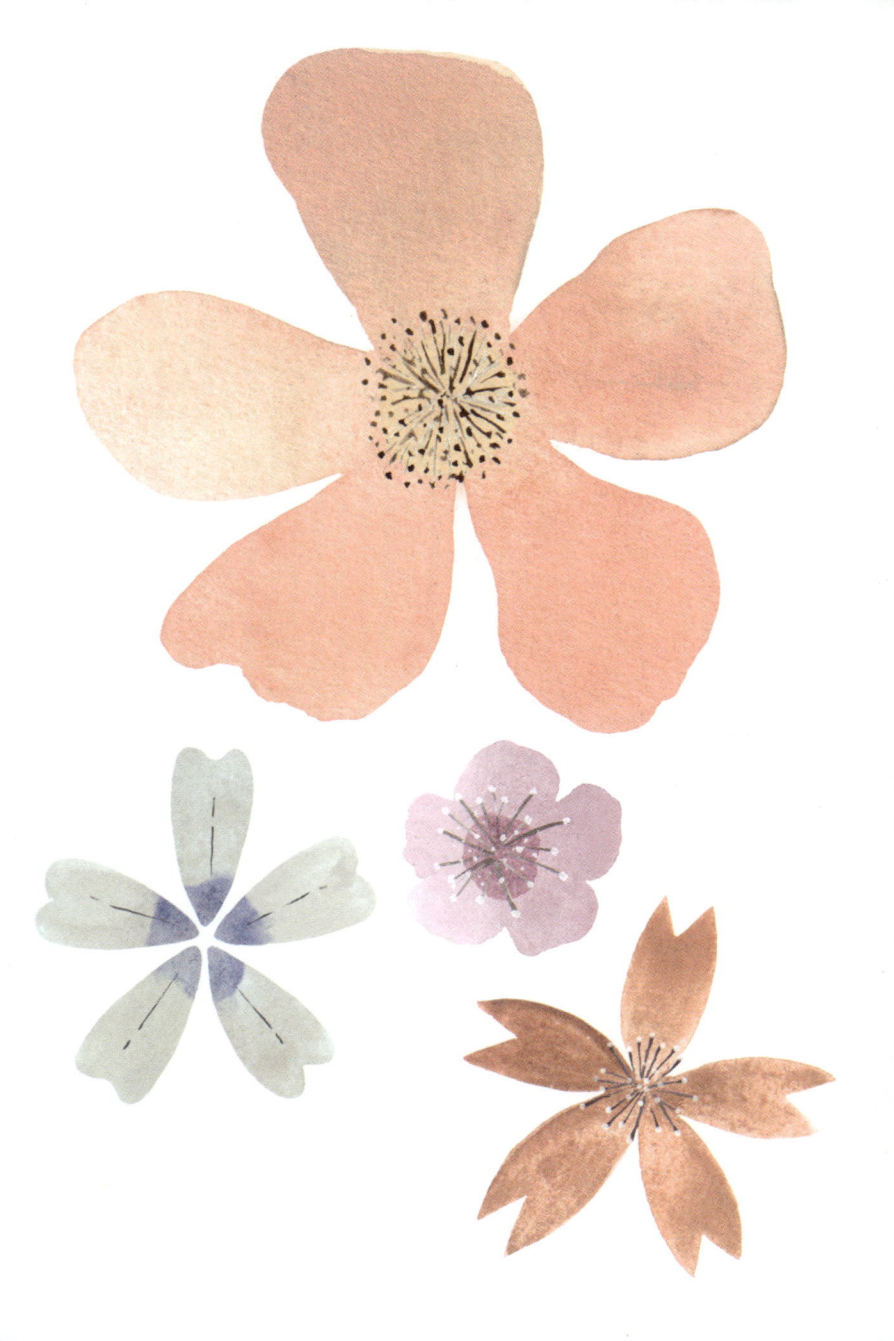

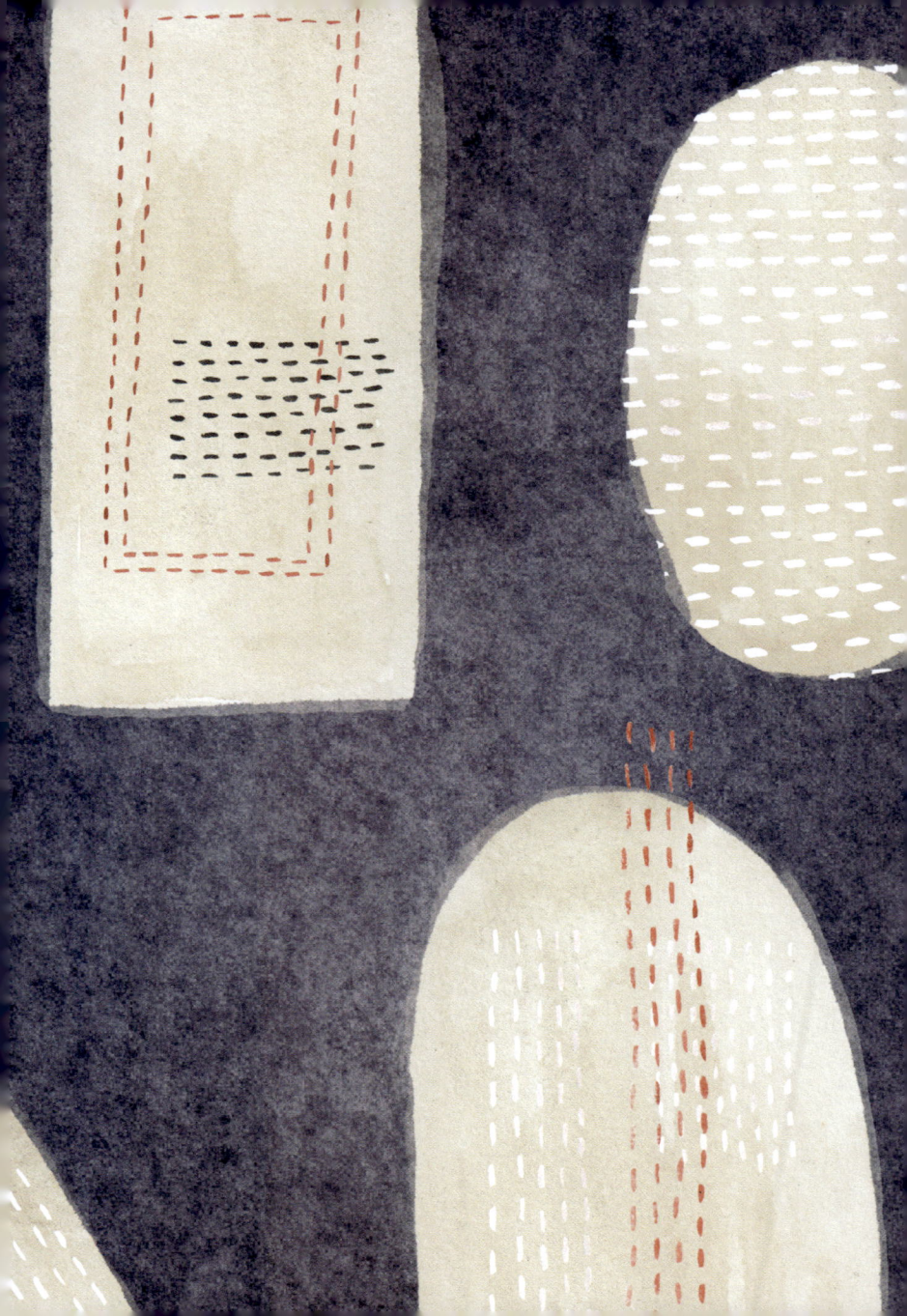

IMPERFECT BEAUTY

JAPANESE CULTURE OFTEN TENDERLY accepts the aging of things. Crafts such as *sashiko* (embroidery), *boro/tsugihagi* (mending textiles), and *kintsugi* (mending broken pottery) focus on giving new life to broken or damaged items. Simple sashiko stitches transform torn and threadbare textiles. Boro and tsugihagi developed from patchworking sashiko-embroidered pieces. In the art of kintsugi, lustrous lacquer bonds and repairs broken pottery fragments, creating lovely designs born from the damage.

Wabi-sabi and shibui form part of an overarching ethos of celebrating so-called flaws and include these mending practices. Wabi-sabi is the Japanese idea of finding beauty in imperfection; shibui offers a similar viewpoint of appreciating beauty in maturity, simplicity, and subtlety. They are both slow by nature and encourage a deep awareness. They say, "Let's not hide our worn, fragmented, imperfect selves. Instead let's attend to the parts that can be mended and refined and make them even more exquisite."

What would it look like to do that for our aging human selves?

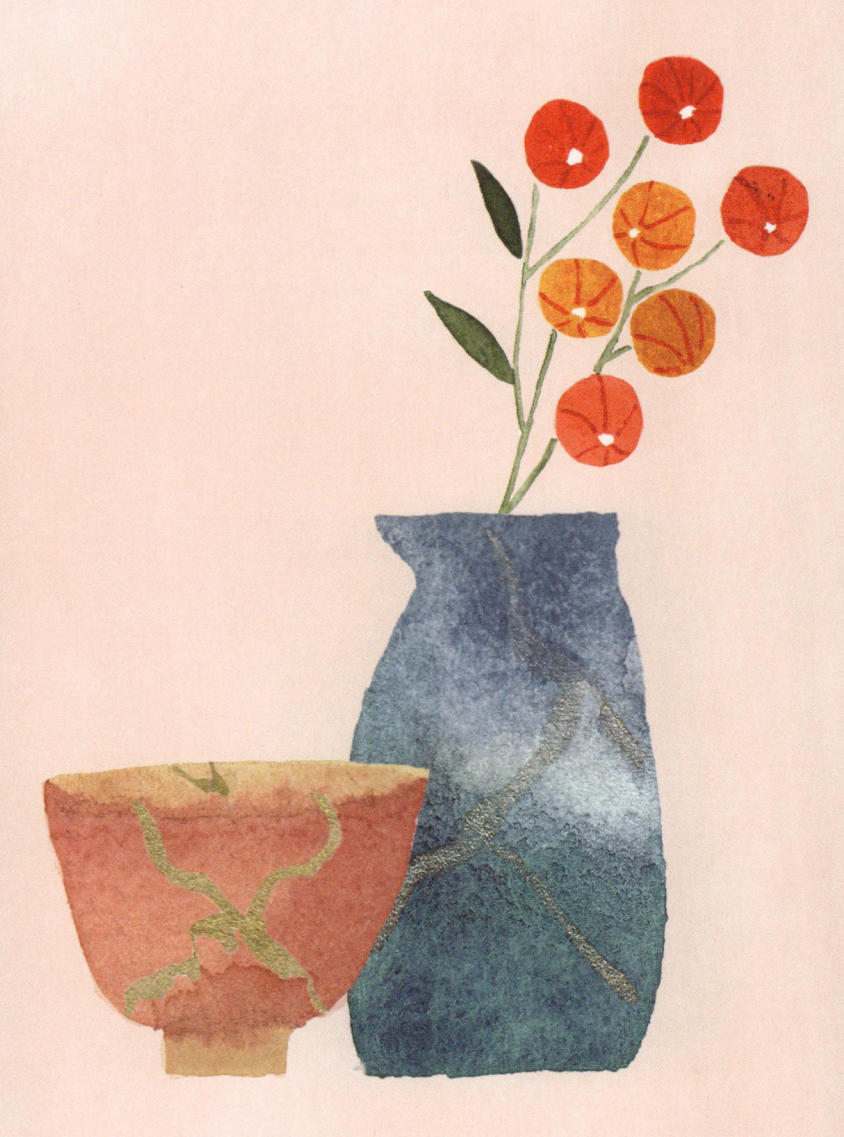

Japanese Crafts

KINTSUGI: An ancient Japanese technique for mending broken pottery using a natural lacquer sourced from *urushi* tree resin. Broken fragments are bonded together with urushi lacquer and flour, and then gold powder is buffed over the glued sections.

SASHIKO: Estimated to have originated in the sixteenth century in Japanese fishing villages, sashiko began as a simple way of mending with running stitches. Daily labor was hard on precious fabric, requiring frequent mending. Over time, the running stitches created distinct patterns that evolved into the beloved embroidery craft.

BORO/TSUGIHAGI: Boro means tattered or repaired, and tsugihagi is a patchwork of scraps. Sashiko stitches frequently hold together and embellish boro and tsugihagi pieces.

Imagine if we approached our aging selves with the same tender acceptance as these Japanese crafts. What if we viewed our wrinkles as golden seams of kintsugi, each line a testament to our experiences and resilience? Our graying or thinning hair as the subtle, mindful stitches of sashiko, silver sparkles reflecting hard-won wisdom? Using these crafts as inspiration, we could fondly piece together the patchwork of our lives—the careers we've had, the roles we've played, the loves we've known. By treating ourselves with the same care and reverence as these cherished objects, we transform the "flaws" of aging into a meaningful panoply of lived experience.

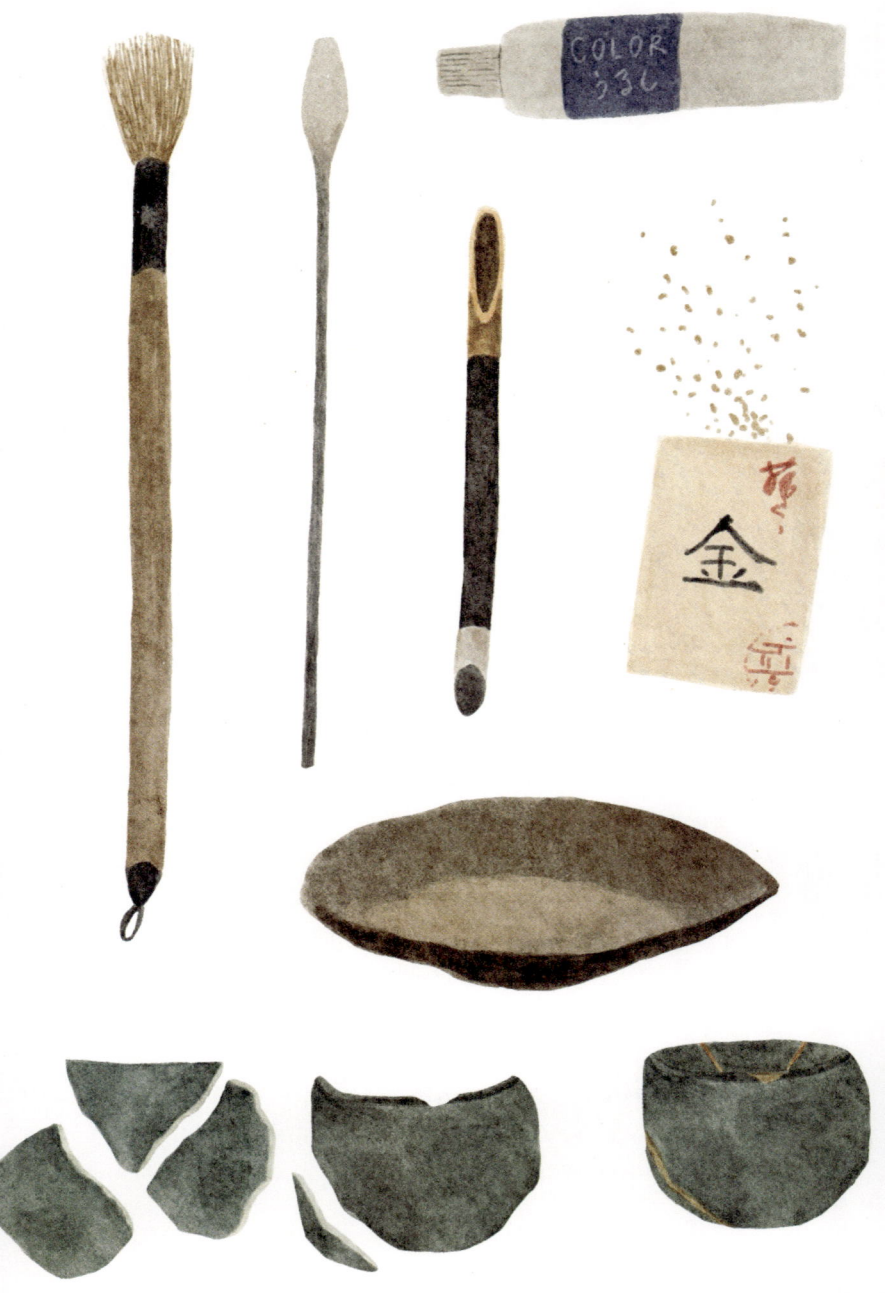

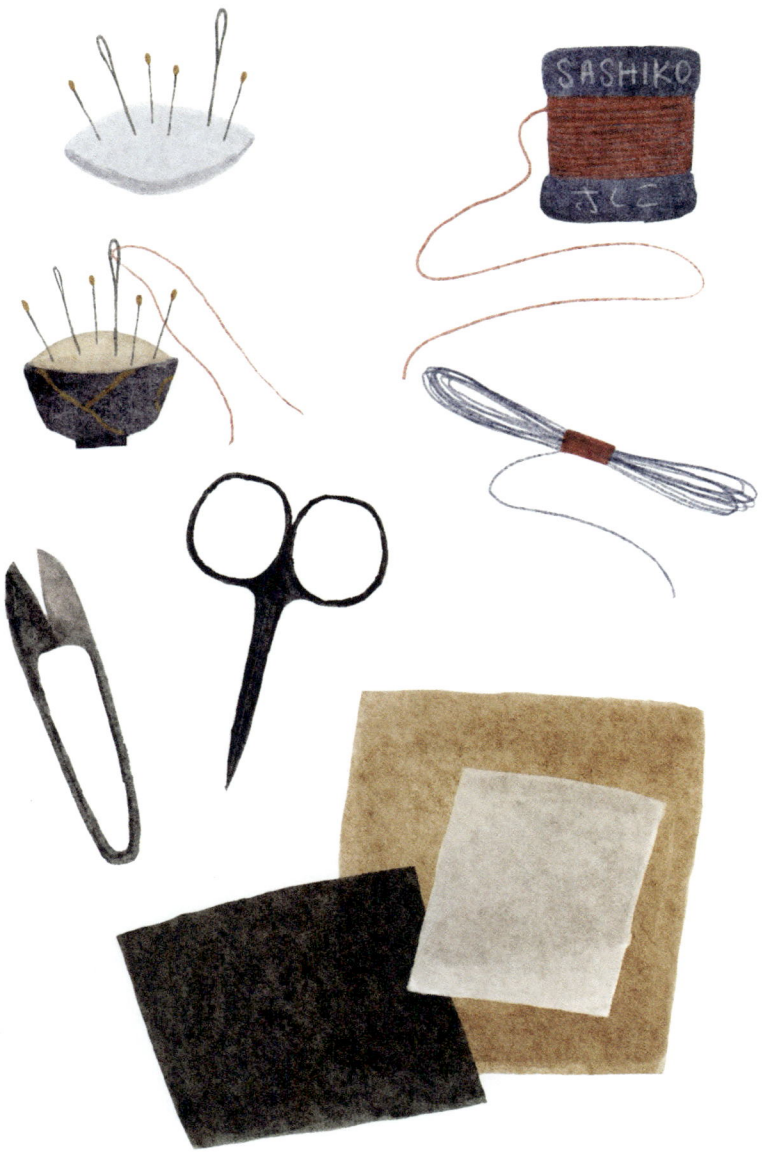

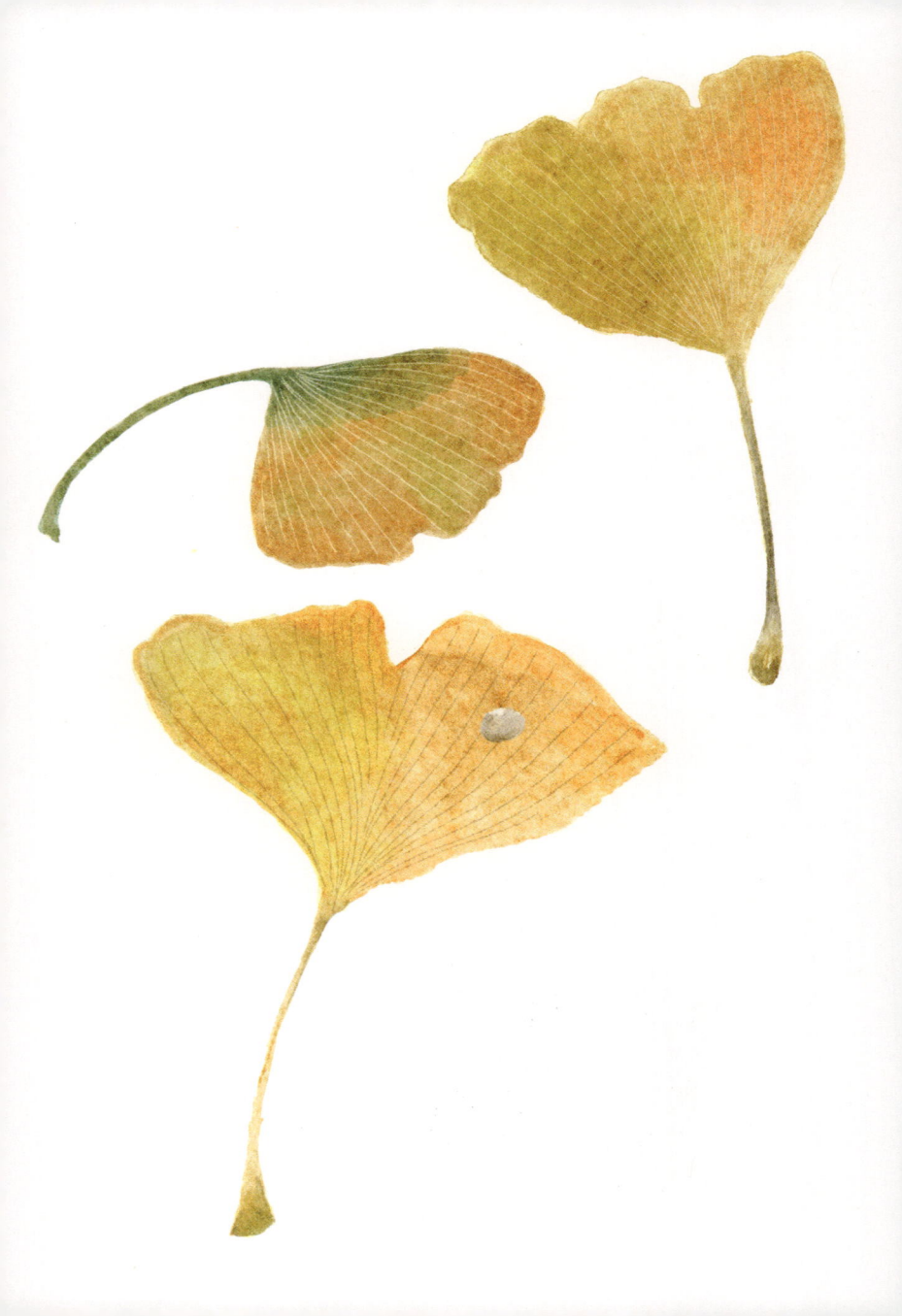

HOW LONG UNTIL
A BEAUTIFUL PLACE?

I WALK EVERY DAY for at least an hour. One day, on a stroll along Seattle's Burke-Gilman Trail, I crossed paths with a woman about my age. "Chinese?" she asked me in heavily accented English. I shook my head and gave her an apologetic smile. She continued in English, "How long until a beautiful place?" We had trouble understanding each other, and I couldn't tell if she was trying to get to a specific location. Frustrated, she trudged off. I stood in the same spot for a while after she left and looked out toward Lake Union. *But we're already in a beautiful place right here,* I thought.

Isn't that how we all live, though? We think that being somewhere else, being someone else, or doing something other than what we're doing will somehow be better. What if we're looking at it all the wrong way?

Just as we may overlook the beauty of our immediate surroundings, we often dismiss the unique charm of late bloomers. This is true in nature and in life. The Japanese concept of *osozaki* reminds us that beauty isn't confined to expected locations or seasons.

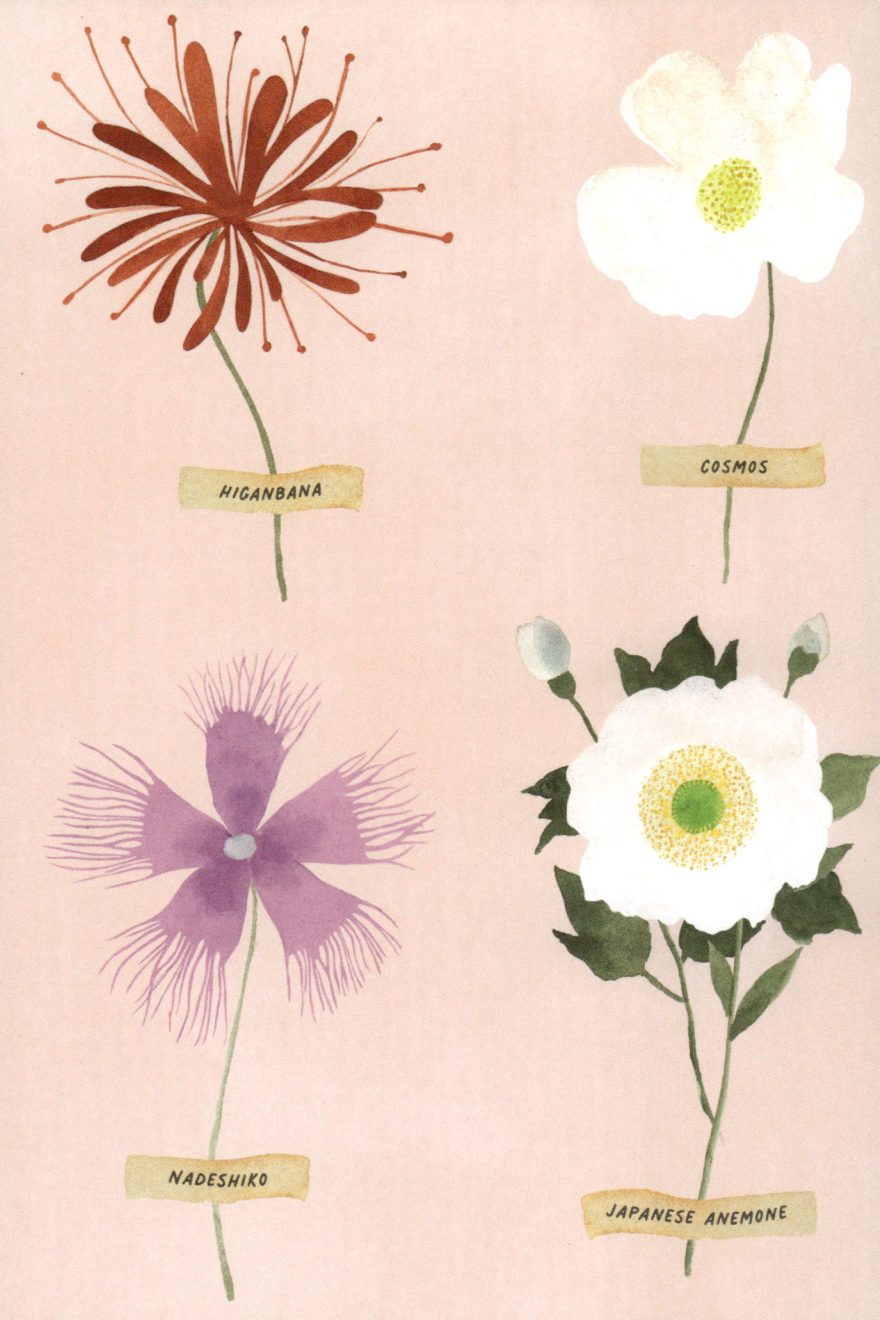

HIGANBANA

COSMOS

NADESHIKO

JAPANESE ANEMONE

Osozaki

Osozaki means "late or slow blooms" in Japanese. I have a special fondness for late bloomers, probably because I've always been one myself. This goes for actual flora, not just people. Sure the effervescence of spring flowers will steal the nature show—who can remain unmoved by the festive cherry blossoms that pop-pop-pop like elegant fireworks to herald the beginning of spring? But as intoxicating as spring blooms are, I particularly admire autumn bloomers such as cosmos and anemones. And, of course, autumnal leaves easily hold their own against springtime flowers. (I also love snowdrops, intrepidly braving the colder temperatures of late winter.) With every year tacked onto this body of mine, I savor slowing down and noticing the permutations of each season. The boldness of spring is a sheer delight, but there's something about the quiet resilience of osozaki that I find endearing. Here are some beautiful Japanese late bloomers and their unique qualities:

HIGANBANA (spider lily or magic lily) has medicinal properties and is used to treat Alzheimer's disease.

COSMOS means simplicity, joy, and beauty.

NADESHIKO (Dianthus superbus) is associated with feminine beauty.

JAPANESE ANEMONES are often used in funerals; these flowers are considered "flowers of the dead."

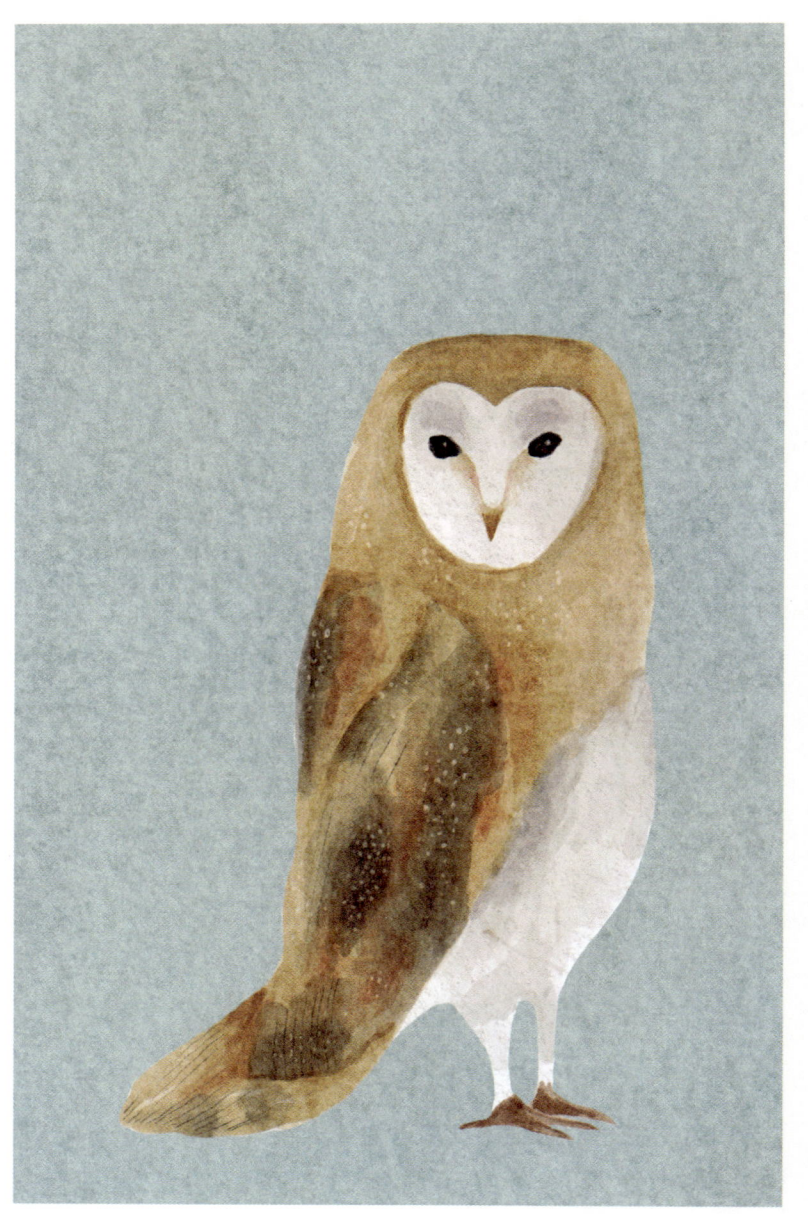

WINSOME WISDOM

THE ASSUMPTION IS THAT as we age, we automatically become wiser. I've been questioning this. I have known both decidedly un-sagacious octogenarians and Yoda-esque tweens. What is wisdom, anyway? For one, it's not merely an accumulation of experiences and observations but an ability to glean life-enhancing perspectives from them.

As a youngster, I defaulted to self-pity. *Why don't I look like Barbie? Why did I end up with immigrant parents? Why is everything so hard?* My theme song would have been titled "Oh woe, why me?" Luckily later in life I started asking myself, *How is this happening FOR me?* Game changer. Instead of viewing circumstances from a victimized stance, I started to see how adversity could be like mental dumbbells or emotional burpees.

The deeply wise consistently remember what we all sort of already know in order to live well: taking care of our health and our loved ones (including the planet), practicing our strengths and befriending our shortcomings, and knowing that our days are numbered, so we might as well exist with as little regret as possible. Wisdom beautifies. It eases us into our true self and adds a twinkle of mischievous wit in our eyes that is unmistakably shibui.

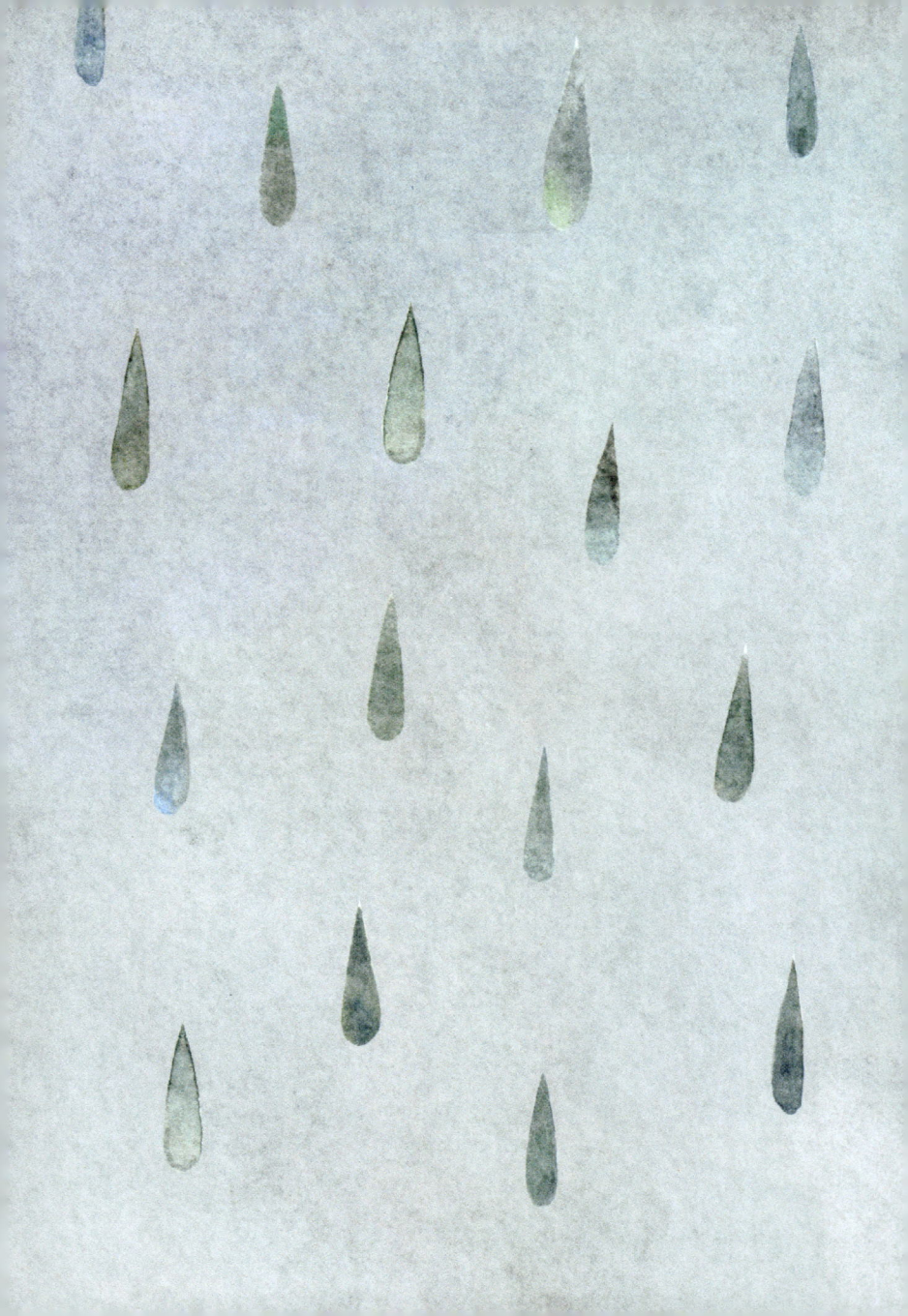

FIRST (IN) SIGHT

I HAD A FLASH of insight at the grocery store one day.

I was shifting impatiently from one foot to the other as an elderly clerk ponderously looked up the prices for my produce items in a small spiral-bound book with laminated pages. He appeared to be in his seventies and was completely oblivious to my deeply meaningful stares, willing him to hurry up. Behind me another clerk was chatting with his customer.

"Until I was twenty, I didn't know that I needed glasses," the clerk behind me said. "I just thought the world was supposed to look kind of fuzzy, sort of ugly and indistinct. Then a friend suggested I might want to get some glasses. So I went to the optometrist around the corner, and I'll never forget it. When I put them on for the first time, I could see everything! It was raining, and I could see the raindrops clearly, as well as every leaf on the trees and all the petals on the flowers—even the stamens. I burst into tears. I didn't know the world was so beautiful. We forget that, don't we?"

Just then the elderly clerk placed the last item into my bag. Was it my imagination, or had he taken his time on purpose? He looked up, smiled, and winked. I smiled back.

Kenshō is a Buddhist term for "first insight," or "initial awakening," or even "seeing one's true nature." Enlightenment-lite, if you will. As I get older and move at a slower pace, I find that I notice more, see more, have more kenshō moments. Truly seeing the depth and breadth of anything or anyone is to recognize beauty. When I'm focused on a craft such as sewing, each stitch becoming a gorgeous tableau in and of itself, I experience everything anew—not just visually but holistically. I am awash with the interwovenness of every fiber in this world.

WRINKLE READING

WRINKLES, LIKE SHIBUI, SPEAK in subtle implications. An aged face tells silent stories—such as a vintage window whose scuffs and scratches whisper of winter storms, harsh sunlight, children at play, and countless other moments, all written in the language of time.

I once stood in front of a giant palm-reading sign comparing my own palm lines to the ones depicted. I was disappointed that my success line was non-existent, but my longevity line looked promising.

Just as palm reading claims to reveal our futures, I've found that wrinkle reading offers insights into a person's past and present. I've studied the faces of older people, and each tells a different life story.

The jovial bunch of senior citizens I tutored in Japan had faces covered with delicate epidermal latticework. They were jokesters, every one of them, and I loved seeing the well-worn grooves enveloping their chortling mugs. A near century of mirth made them look like ancient Shar Pei dogs.

Then there was that vivacious woman in a café. She was probably at least a decade older than me, and my first thought was, *I want to be like her when I grow up!*

As she chatted with her friend, her crow's feet winked from behind stylish glasses, and her ever-changing countenance created fascinating patterns of expression lines. A constantly shifting cartography of an engaged life. Her confidence lit up everything around her.

Through wrinkle reading, I've begun to pick up on the ones who have a merry outlook on life, the ones who have suffered immensely, the ones whose lines have calcified into an expression of rage, and even the ones who've been cosmetically altered. Once, in a West Hollywood grocery store, I brushed past a woman who'd had so much work done that she looked like the dreaded "after" photo of plastic surgeries gone wrong. It seemed that in her effort to banish all signs of aging, she'd lost some of her humanity.

As I trace the emerging lines on my own face, I see them through the lens of shibui. I view my forehead wrinkles as surprise lines rather than frown lines—or perhaps curiosity lines from insatiable inquisitiveness. I've grown to adore my crow's feet that are evidence of laughter and a life fully lived. In embracing these changes, I'm discovering the deep, subtle beauty that only time can create.

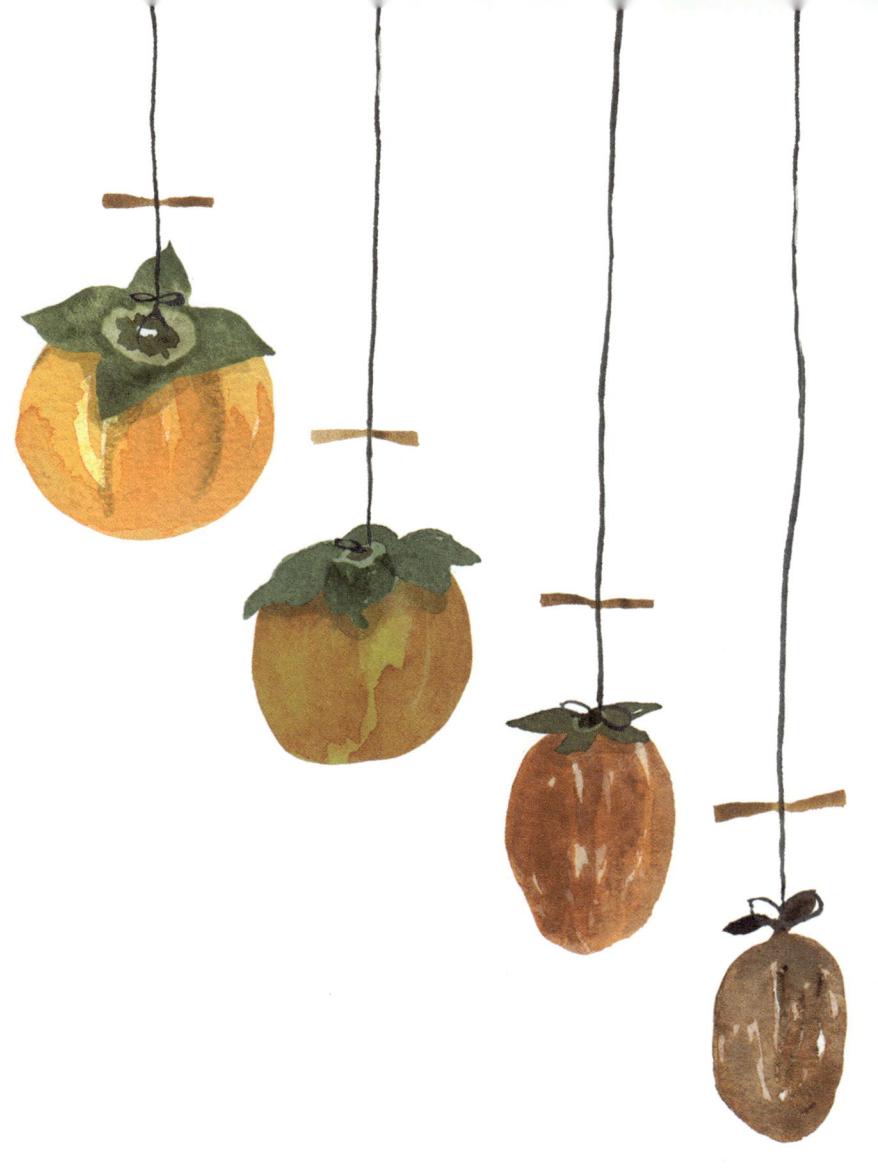

TO MAKE HOSHIGAKI, PERSIMMONS ARE AIR-DRIED FOR
SEVERAL WEEKS. THEY TASTE A LITTLE LIKE DRIED DATES.

The Alchemy of Tea

The Japanese word for tea is *cha*. A true superfood rich in antioxidants, green tea has an impressive list of benefits:

- Reduces anxiety and stress
- May protect against cognitive decline
- Supports bone health
- Improves health span and longevity
- Lowers cholesterol
- May enhance memory
- May manage and prevent type 2 diabetes
- Lowers risk of heart disease and strokes
- Reduces high blood pressure

Tea is purported to have been brought from China to Japan by a Zen Buddhist monk around 800 CE. There are more than twenty varieties of Japanese green tea, which is sweeter than Chinese variations, though both produce deliciously vegetal and slightly astringent and bitter (shibui!) undertones. I took part in many tea ceremonies when I lived in Japan, and I particularly enjoyed the communal aspect of sharing a gigantic bowl of freshly brewed matcha with other attendees. We would take a sip, rotate the bowl slightly, and then pass it to the next person. It was an intimate and calming experience. I have multiple cups of green tea every day and like to make my own blends. Tea is a magical concoction that enhances beauty in every way.

SENCHA

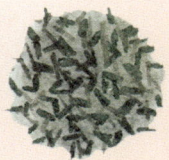

From the first harvest. Very mild with a little bit of caffeine.

MATCHA

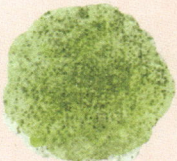

Powdered tencha leaves. Bright green and has more caffeine.

HŌJICHA

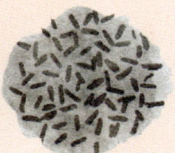

Roasted green tea leaves. Very little caffeine with a rich, earthy taste.

BANCHA

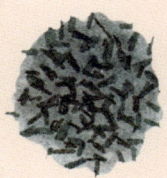

From the second harvest of the same plant as sencha, but with larger leaves.

GENMAICHA

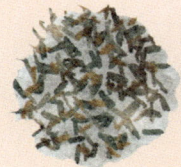

Sencha plus roasted rice. Nutty with sesame-like flavor. Less caffeine.

TENCHA

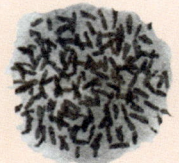

Purest form of green tea leaves without veins, stems, stalks, etc.

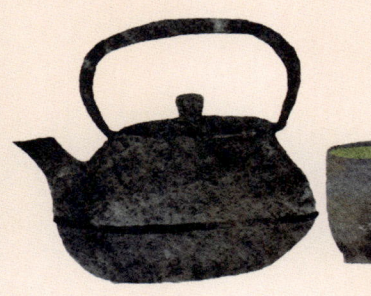

FAVORITE BLENDS:

Honeybush + hōjicha + hemp milk

Sencha + nettle tea

Matcha + roasted dandelion tea + hemp milk

Cacao shell tea + hōjicha

病は気から
Yamai wa ki kara (Sickness and health start with the mind)

A JAPANESE PROVERB

健康

Kenkō

HEALTH

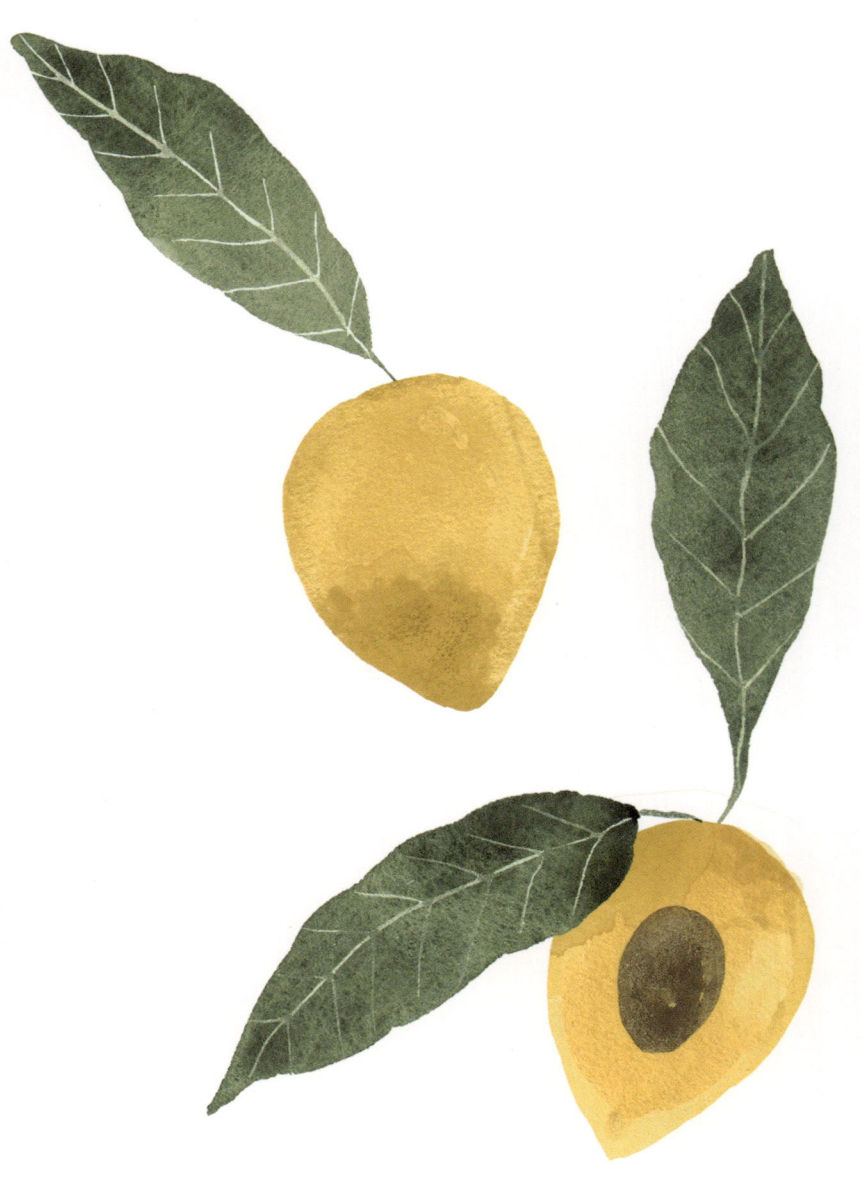

LOQUATS HAVE MANY HEALTH BENEFITS, ESPECIALLY THE LEAVES.

ON VITALITY

WHEN I WAS DIAGNOSED with an overactive thyroid in 2012, my Harvard-trained endocrinologist prescribed hormone suppressants and advised that I surgically remove my thyroid. I'm no physician, but I knew at a profound level that treating the symptoms with meds or cutting out an organ wasn't the right solution for me. My doctor expressed her reservations, but she agreed to let me follow my instincts. I chose a path aligned with shibui principles: trusting nature and appreciating my body's wisdom. By caring for my whole self—mind, body, and spirit—I've managed my condition for well over a decade. This experience has taught me that health, like shibui beauty, emerges from within and deepens with time and attention.

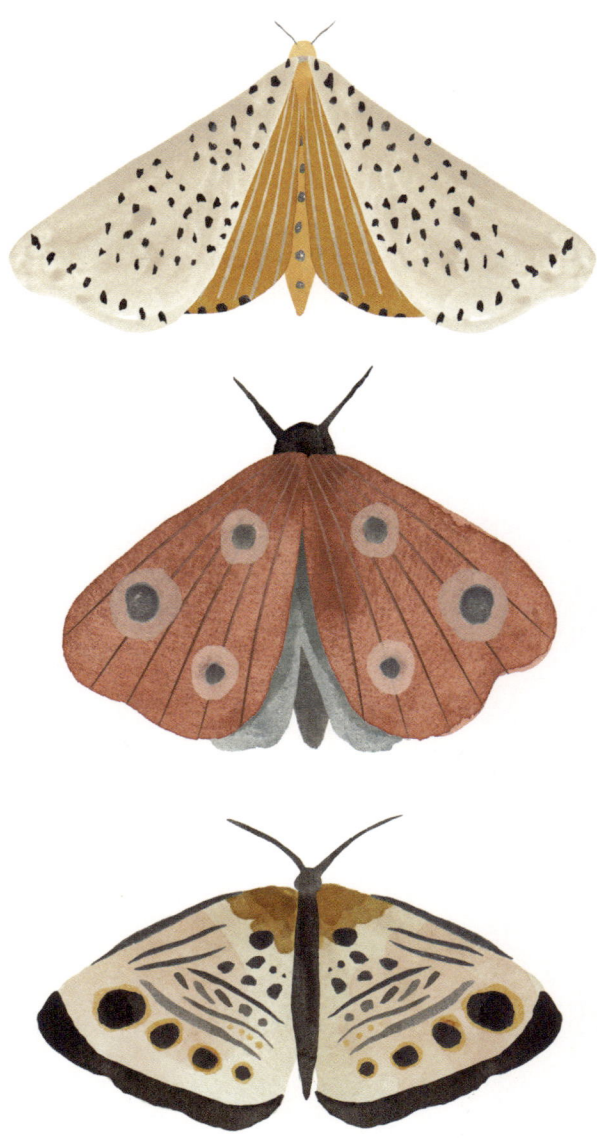

THE JOY OF MENOPAUSE

WHEN I WAS IN my early thirties, my mother told me that she'd gone through *kōnenki* (menopause) at thirty-eight years old. This alarmed me, as marriage and babies weren't yet on my horizon, and I unequivocally wanted both. When pressed for details, she made menopause sound like a non-issue, casually waving it off with "Good riddance."

Two decades later, my own menopausal rite of passage arrived at the standard age of fifty-two. Like my mother's experience, it passed with little disruption, and I assumed it was the same for most women. I had no clue.

In the United States, menopause isn't a comfortable milestone to examine. Like letting our hair go gray, the topic seems taboo, even among women. Sure there's the exaggerated fanning of the face with "Ugh, hot flashes!" or a mocking lament about night sweats, but rarely have I had a candid conversation about this momentous time in a woman's life. This seems strange to me.

Japanese women, in contrast, seem to speak more openly about kōnenki, considering it a time of renewal and rebirth—an embodiment of the shibui principle of finding beauty in life's transitions. Rather than viewing menopause as an ending, they see it as a transformation in which our experiences crystallize into wisdom and revived purpose.

And indeed I feel more powerful. I've experienced a surge in self-esteem. Self-doubt and other people's opinions slide off me like eggs on nonstick cookware (okay perhaps not *always*, but most of the time). Qualities that seemed so elusive in my twenties, thirties, and even forties are now anchoring characteristics. And what freedom it is to no longer worry about premenstrual mood swings or breakouts or sullied clothes and bedding. Perhaps the problem lies in the name: menopause. It suggests we're on pause once we can no longer conceive. What if we call it kōnenki instead and celebrate this time of renewed growth and possibilities?

Breathe

I have read countless meditation and mindfulness books on breathing exercises. Yet I rarely think of breathing as nourishment. A method to calm a palpitating heart or racing mind, yes. A necessary function for living, obviously.

I don't breathe deeply enough—I know this—and I've been working on changing my breathing habits.

Here are some helpful breathing techniques you can incorporate without a formal meditation practice:

- Inhale for three counts, hold for four counts, and exhale for five counts.
- Touch the tip of your tongue to the back of your two front teeth and breathe deeply in and out ten times with your mouth closed.
- When you wake up in the morning, take one deep breath and assess how your body feels. Notice, then let go. Repeat at bedtime.

Conscious breathing is a quintessentially shibui practice. Perhaps *the* most essential part of being human, the breath is readily available, and with consistent practice, the benefits of conscious breathing increase as our organs age. It connects us to the present moment and helps us appreciate the simple and remarkable act of being alive.

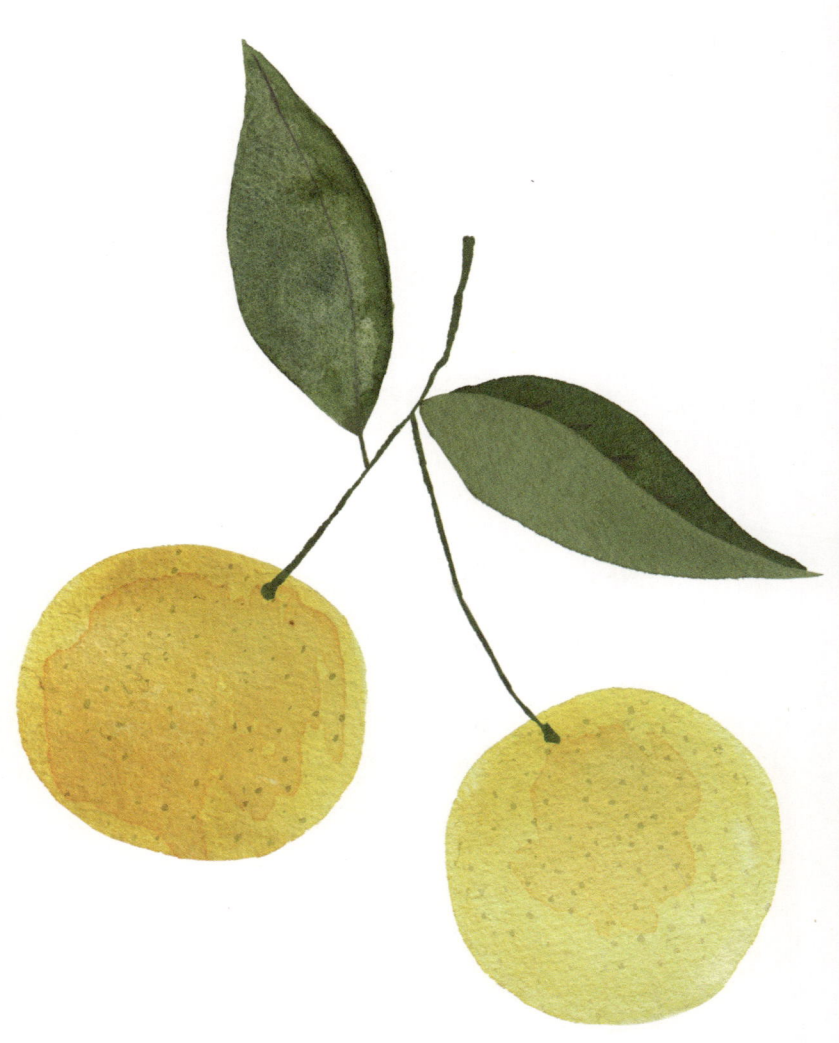

yuzu

THE BENEFITS OF RESTRAINT

HARA HACHI BU REFERS to eating up to 80 percent fullness—not to stuff yourself silly, but rather to eat just until you're no longer hungry. This ancient Japanese precept is challenging for most people. We are flooded with infinite options for delectable food. And not only food! Everything is just a click away. Fighting the temptation to overconsume can feel like a losing battle.

Hara hachi bu has plenty of benefits: not only does it reduce the likelihood of weight gain and its associated ailments, but you are also more conscious of each bite— more aware of the taste and texture of the food.

Imagine applying this mindful approach to other areas of consumption. What if you only spent 80 percent of your allotted budget? Or similarly constrained screen time? In this modern era of too many choices, is it possible that hara hachi bu is the key to better living?

The idea of hara hachi bu taps into shibui wisdom. By moderating our expectations and accepting natural changes, we can find greater contentment. Just as stopping at 80 percent fullness leaves room for digestion, tuning into our aging process with grace allows space for new experiences and personal growth.

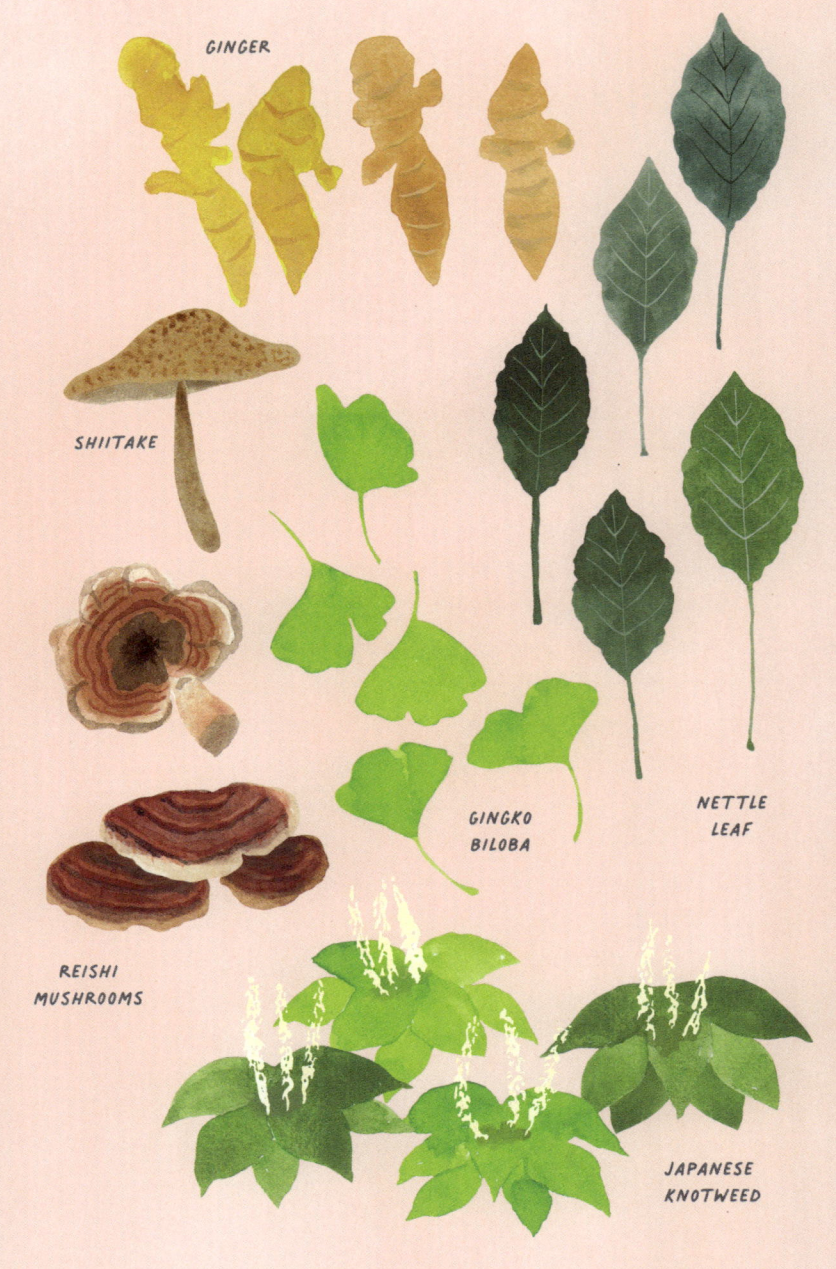

GINGER

SHIITAKE

NETTLE
LEAF

GINGKO
BILOBA

REISHI
MUSHROOMS

JAPANESE
KNOTWEED

Ancient Japanese Herbs and Healing Practices

Eastern medicine focuses on preventative health measures. *Kampō* is a Japanese healing practice that originated in Chinese medicine, in which herbs are widely used, often steeped as tea or consumed as broths or soups.

NETTLE LEAVES are typically served as tea at the end of the winter to prevent allergies.

GINGER is incorporated into many dishes and is touted for its anti-inflammatory properties.

JAPANESE KNOTWEED, hailed for its anti-inflammatory and antioxidant qualities, is particularly effective for cardiovascular issues and joint pain.

SHIITAKE AND REISHI MUSHROOMS, though currently trendy, have been superheroes in the kampō sphere for thousands of years. They promote mental acuity, heightened focus, and immune system support.

GINGKO BILOBA is ingested as an herbal supplement and is said to enhance memory and cognition and improve circulation and eye health. The gingko biloba tree is native to many Asian countries.

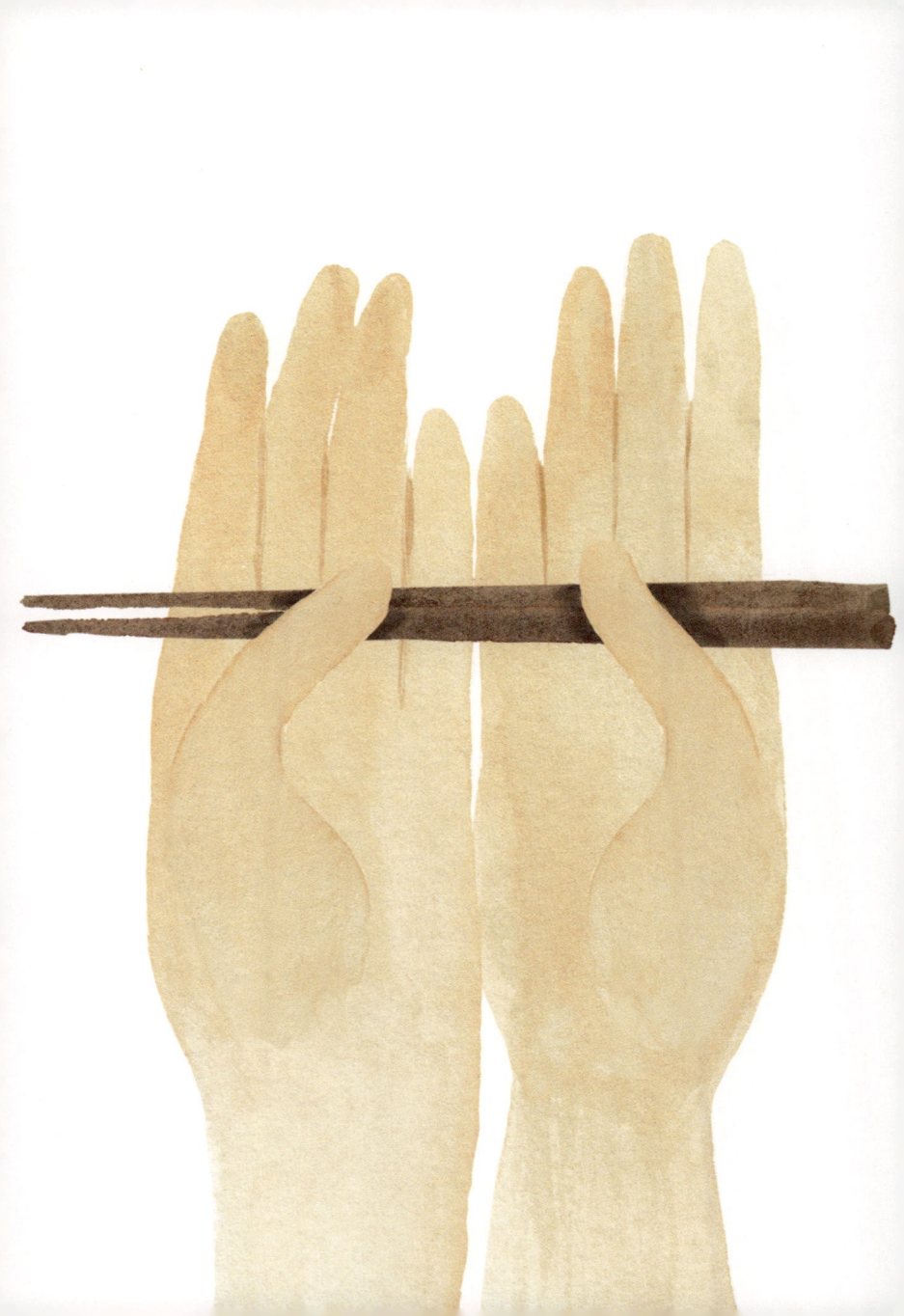

PUT YOUR HANDS TOGETHER

JAPANESE PEOPLE AREN'T GENERALLY considered religious in the way communities in other parts of the world identify with one faith or another. Japanese culture seems to embody the oft-touted phrase, "I'm not religious, but I *am* spiritual." A mashup of Shintō and Buddhism and even some Judeo-Christian ideologies pepper the Japanese lifestyle. Decorated trees pop up for Christmas in most parts of Japan, the New Year is celebrated at Shintō shrines, and Buddhist tea ceremonies are performed on various occasions throughout the year.

If there is a type of faith aligned with the Japanese, gratitude might be it. Every meal starts with putting the hands together and saying, "*Itadakimasu*," a declaration of thanks for the food, directly translated as "I humbly receive," but with a sense of festivity and bon appétit.

After a meal, the hands kiss again with the utterance of "*Gochisōsama*," meaning "thank you for the meal" or "it was a feast!" What a wonderful devotional act.

Cultivating gratitude becomes even more poignant as our lifespans shorten. The beautiful Japanese practice of expressing thanks could bookend each day. *Thank you for this life. I humbly accept. What a smorgasbord!*

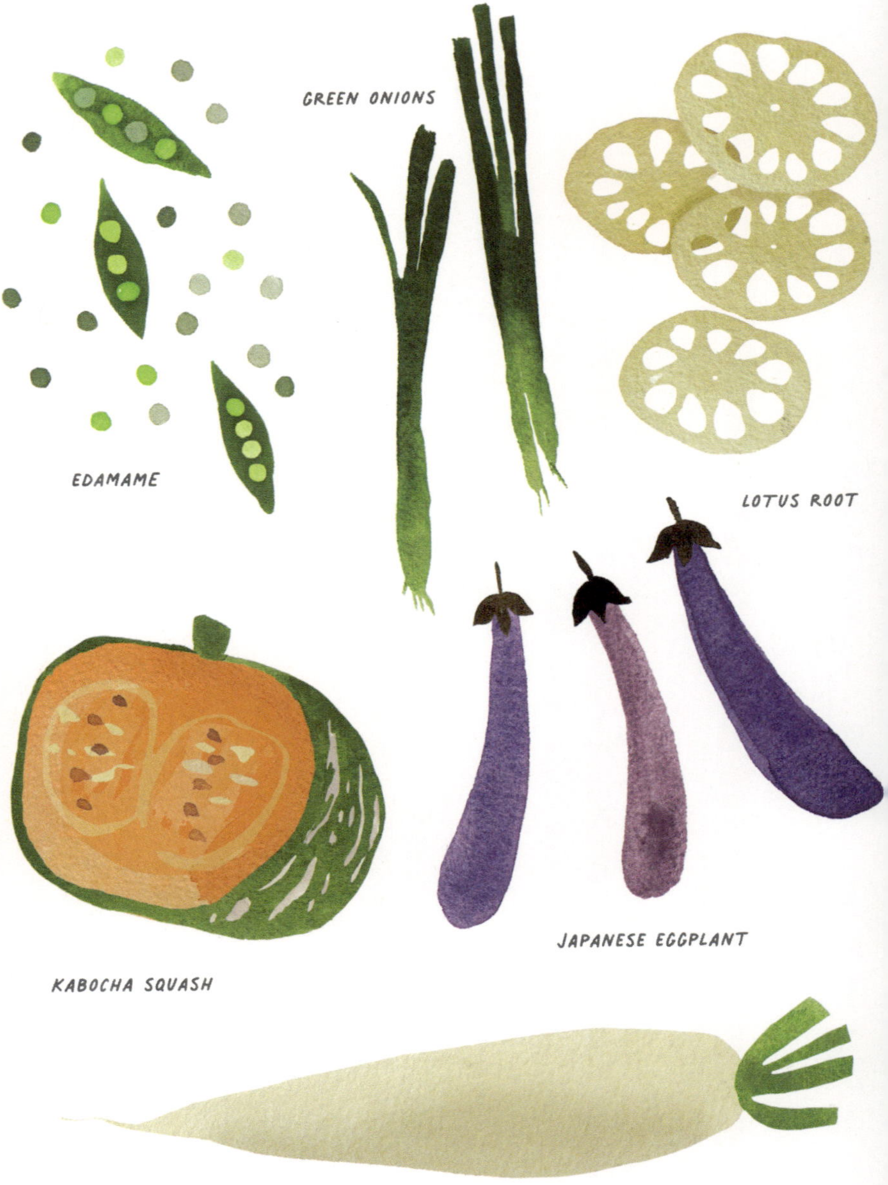

GREEN ONIONS

EDAMAME

LOTUS ROOT

KABOCHA SQUASH

JAPANESE EGGPLANT

DAIKON RADISH

NOURISHING THE WHOLE SELF

LIVING WITH AN AUTOIMMUNE condition teaches me the delicate balance our bodies maintain. During the pandemic, prolonged stress triggered a severe gum disease flare-up, and I lost a molar. Rather than despairing, I followed a holistic approach to healing, cutting out all sugar and processed foods, increasing my exercise, and improving my sleep. Most importantly I worked on trusting my body and its innate ability to heal itself, despite my periodontist telling me that gum disease is irreversible.

The results were remarkable. Within six weeks, my gums showed significant improvement, surprising even my dentist. This experience reinforced a vital lesson: while aging brings inevitable changes, our bodies retain an impressive capacity for renewal when properly nourished.

The Japanese concept of *eiyō* extends beyond mere nutrition to encompass everything that feeds our whole self: physical sustenance, mental stimulation, emotional fulfillment, and spiritual growth. As we age, this whole-self nourishment becomes even more crucial.

My health challenges—including aging itself—are constant reminders of life's fragility and have become a shibui guide, urging me to care for my whole being.

The Magic of Sleepy Time

Sleep, the unsung hero of health maintenance, becomes evermore precious as we age.

Traditional Japanese sleeping involved futon mattresses on tatami mats, though most Japanese now prefer Western-style beds. On a recent trip to Japan, I slept on the floor, tucked between the coziest comforter and a plush futon mattress—blissful until my bed-accustomed back protested the next morning.

While sleeping accommodations matter, I believe the presleep routine is even more important. My own includes:

- Journaling. I like to record all the tasks I accomplished, big and small.
- Taking an evening shower. Washing at night is a Japanese custom symbolizing purification.
- Caring for my skin with simple and nourishing ointments.
- Reading. I try to stay away from heart-pounding thrillers that will keep me awake into the wee hours.

Quality sleep is essential for aging well, in a shibui way. It's when our bodies repair, rejuvenate, and harmonize.

Just like kampō, sleep reflects the shibui approach to health: gentle, natural, everyday interventions that work with the body's wisdom, helping us age with resilience, grace, and harmony.

HOW ARE YOU?

IF YOU HAPPENED UPON an acquaintance or friend in Japan, they would probably ask you, "*Genki desuka?*" or the slightly politer version, "*O genki desuka?*" The greeting asks, "Are you genki?" or the English equivalent of "How are you?"

And just as you would probably respond, "Fine," most Japanese folks will reply, "Genki." But genki is one of those quintessentially Japanese words that is difficult to fully translate into other languages, its connotation too limited for the word "fine." It's a sense of well-being, but it's also a kind of energetic, lively vibe. Genki implies being full of spirit or vitality. *Gen* means "origin" or "source," and *ki* refers to the life force coursing through all of us. I love the word genki—its bright and buoyant nature connects so inherently to the source of breathing, waking, living.

As we age, maintaining our genki becomes both more challenging and more rewarding. Embracing the shibui concept, we can cultivate a deep-rooted vitality that grows richer with time, much like a batch of gut health–boosting *takuan* pickles or a gorgeously weathered piece of wood.

*Like wildflowers, you must allow yourself
to grow in all the places people thought
you never would.*

E.V. ROGINA

目的

Mokuteki

PURPOSE

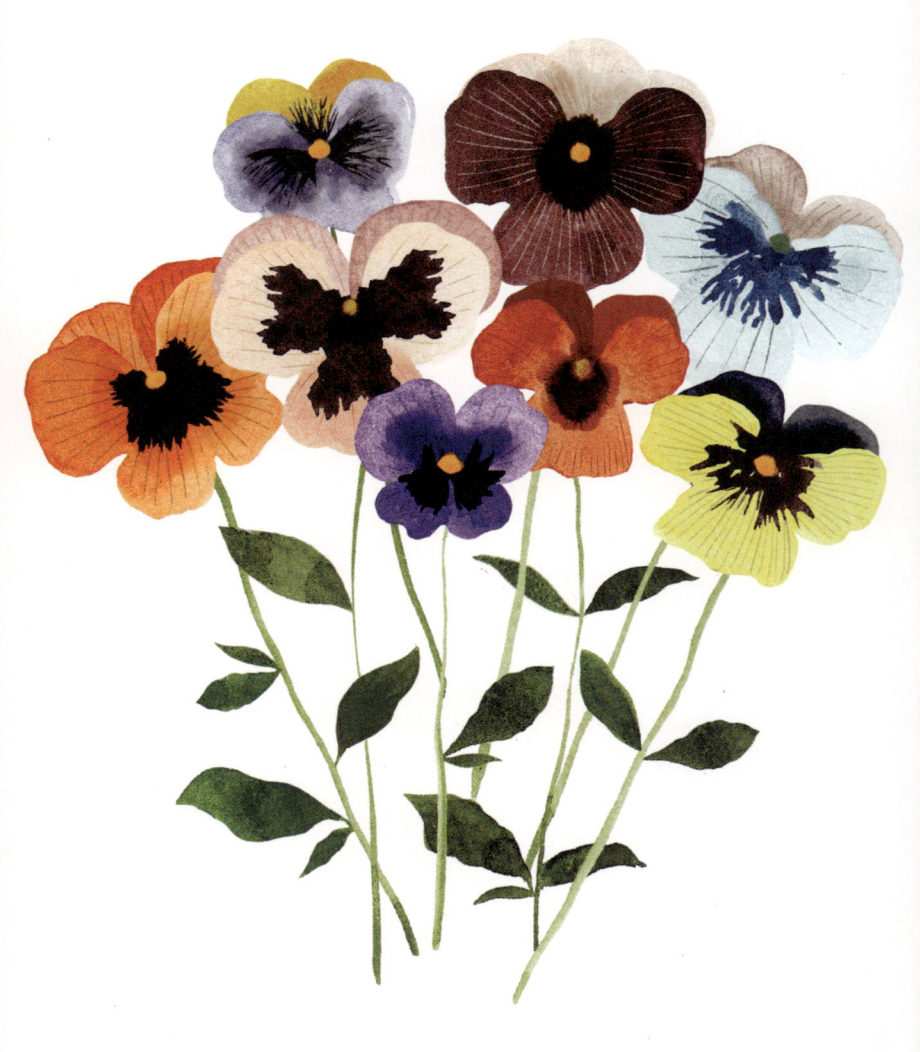

ON PURPOSE

THE JAPANESE CONCEPT OF *ikigai* (a reason for being) has gained popularity, but I find myself more drawn to the humbler notion of *mokuteki* (purpose). If ikigai is an all-night hike up Mount Fuji to see the spectacular sunrise, mokuteki is the daily twenty-minute walk around the neighborhood. This focus on humility and accessibility is a shift in perspective that embodies the essence of shibui.

There's a quiet, understated quality of "everydayness" to all things shibui. Our mokuteki—our daily purposes—need not be grand or publicly declared. They can be as modest as tending a garden or practicing needlecraft. These unassuming, consistent actions align with one of my mother's favorite Japanese proverbs, "*Chiri mo tsumoreba yama to naru*" (even small particles of dust, when accumulated, can become a mountain).

As we grow older, we can find beauty and meaning in everyday mokuteki duties. Tiny, seemingly insignificant actions practiced over time are worthwhile in and of itself. It's a gentle reminder that purpose isn't always about achieving great feats (Earn a million dollars! Become a social media influencer!) but about doing small things with deliberate, intentional, unconditional love.

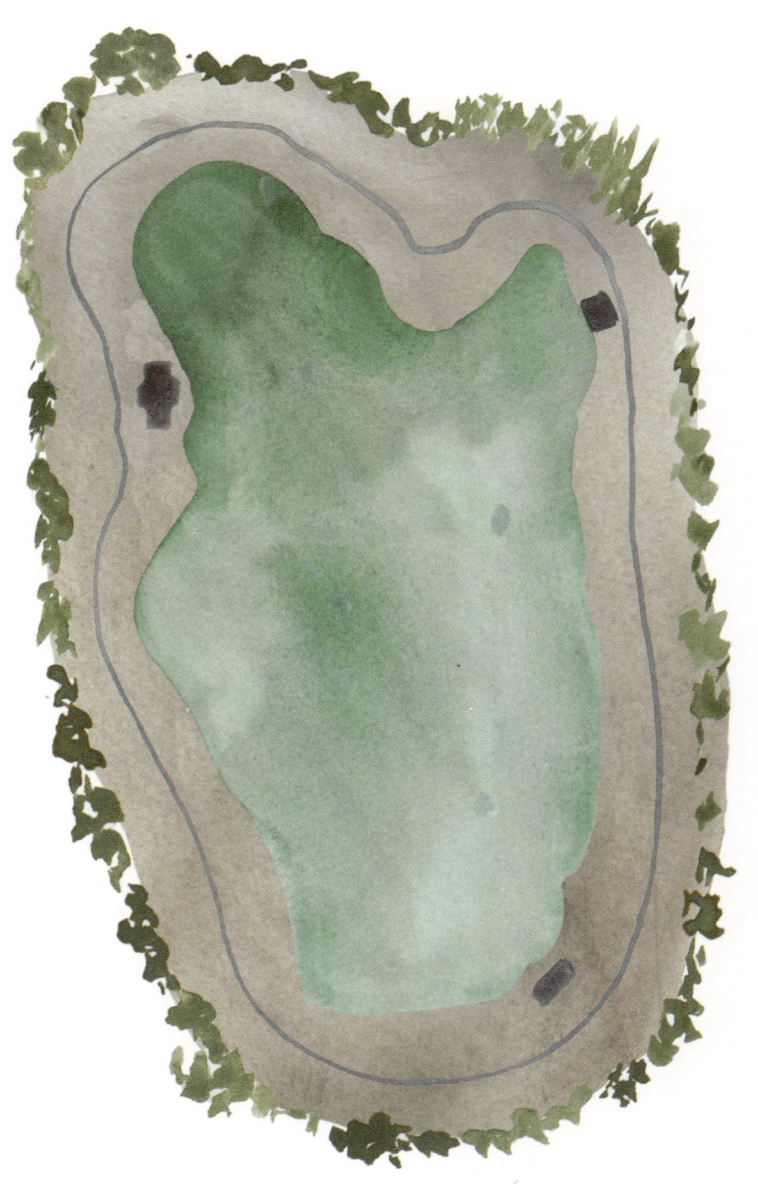

THE GREEN LAKE LOOP

THE LOOP

NEAR MY HOUSE, GREEN LAKE is encircled by a three-mile trail bustling with walkers, runners, cyclists, skaters, pets, and waterfowl. Lush foliage surrounds the path, and true to its name, the lake maintains its suspiciously verdant shade year-round.

My loop strolls have become a metaphor for shibui aging. One day I watched a young dad racing around with a stroller at breakneck speed. I remembered my younger workaholic self, rushing toward what I thought was success—yet like this loop, merely going round and round the same endless path.

In contrast I often see an elderly woman bent double yet moving steadily, her little dog matching her pace. Her gait is painstakingly slow, and she greets everyone with a smile. Speed means so little when there's such joy in simply moving and taking in the view. We rush about more and more . . . but for what?

As I've aged, I meditate on the thought that there really is no "there" there. We're all on this loop of life, and rather than focusing solely on reaching an arbitrary finish line, may we find beauty and meaning in each circuit.

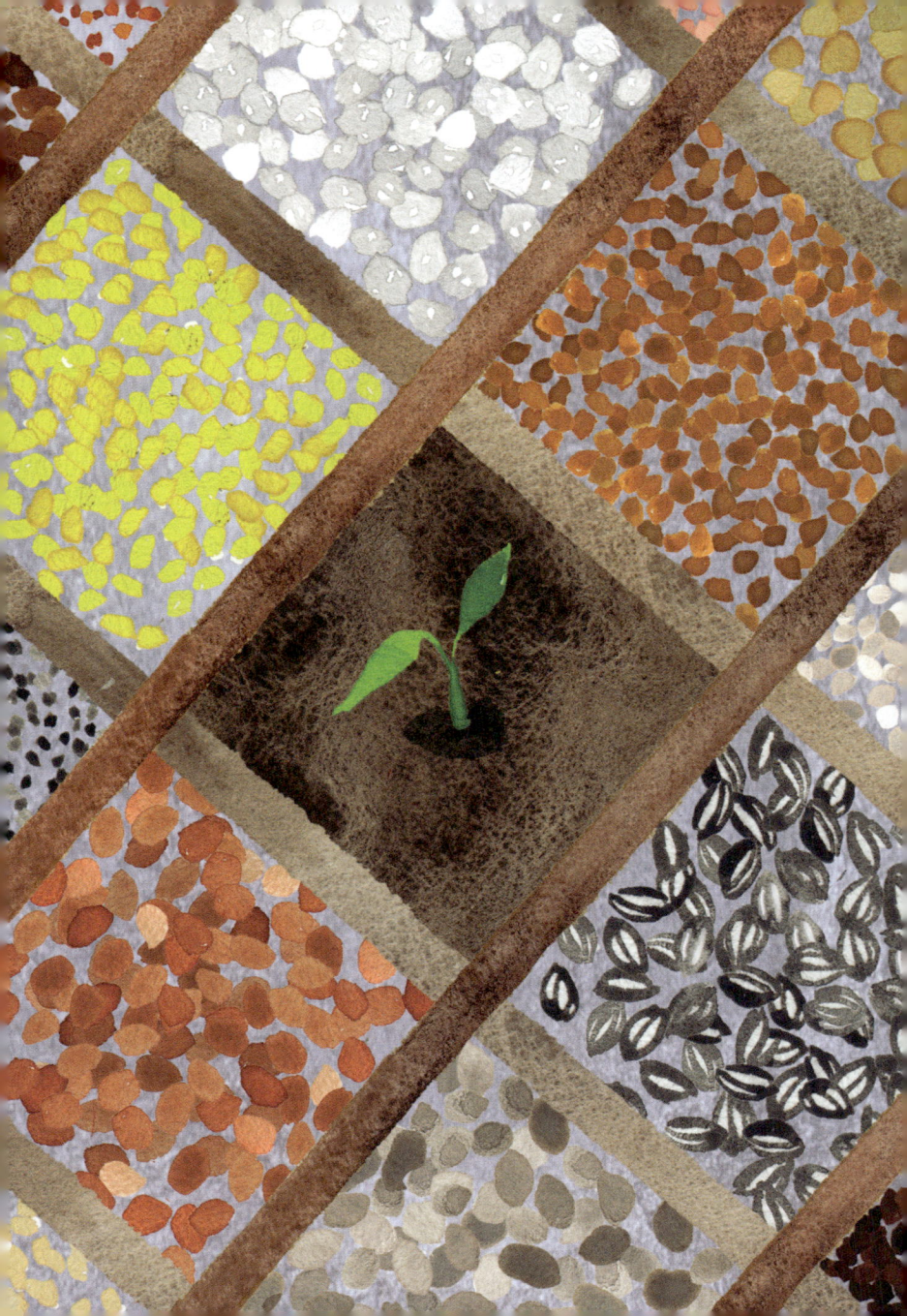

FROM NOTHING TO SOMETHING

ONCE I WAS ASKED, "What is creativity?"

Isn't the whole point of life to create? We give birth to children, ideas, art, gardens, businesses, cities, inventions. After much contemplation, I've settled on, "Creativity is when you intentionally generate something from seemingly nothing." The Japanese word *sōsaku* captures this idea, meaning both creativity and creative *work*.

Society often expects creative output to diminish with advancing age. But the shibui perspective challenges this notion, suggesting that our creativity can flourish and become more nuanced with time.

An investment banker friend once claimed she wasn't creative at all. I hear this too often, a misconception that stems from a narrow definition of creativity, often limited to visual, musical, or written arts. But creativity, like the concept of shibui, is far more encompassing. It's present in how we solve problems, in how we adapt to the changes aging brings, and in how we find new ways to connect with others.

The moment we make nothing into something, we perform a distinctive alchemy, a magic that doesn't dwindle with age. This is the crux of *sōsaku* and it's a vital part of aging with grace and purpose.

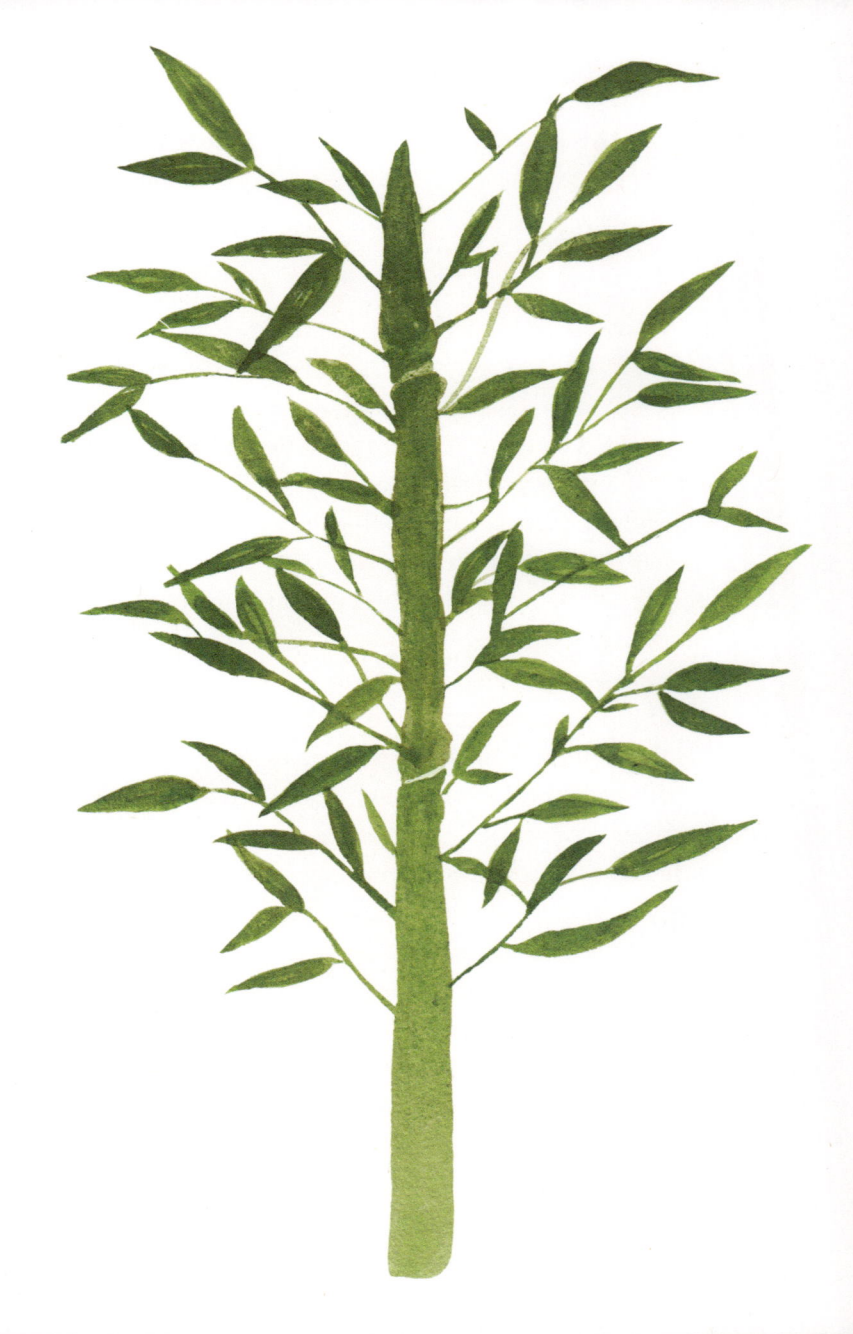

RETIREMENT: REDEFINING PURPOSE IN LATER YEARS

THE WESTERN CONCEPT OF retirement often clashes with the shibui approach to aging. I plan to never retire. At least not in the traditional sense. I love my work. I can't believe that I get to spend my time with pen, paintbrush, and sewing needle in hand, and I would do these things regardless of whether I get a paycheck or not. I hope to be clutching one of my beloved tools when I heave my last breath.

This doesn't mean that I revel in every aspect of my work. Sometimes I grouse, cry, or feel overwhelmed. But in the moments when I settle into a groove, I feel like I'm contributing a useful, unique aspect of myself, and all the negative parts feel worth it. In fact I may even need the negative parts to appreciate the good ones.

Recently I joined a yoga retreat in Mexico with a dear friend and a group of women, mostly in their sixties and seventies. My friend had been practicing yoga for decades, but I'd only dabbled. As you can imagine, I had trouble keeping up with the rigorous yoga sessions, but there were other aspects of the retreat I was immediately drawn to, such as visiting a sumptuous botanical garden, taking a boat ride to an enchanting island for easy hikes and delicious meals, traipsing along the beach, and touring art galleries.

The women were companionable, and the retreat was a charming escape from reality, with exquisitely prepared meals featuring local Mexican ingredients, striking architecture and stunning landscapes, and art and various wares for sale. We were even serenaded by mariachi bands and violinists at luxurious hotel restaurants overlooking the sea.

But when my friend told me, "I don't want to leave," at the end of our six-day stay, I was surprised to realize that I was more than ready to go home. There we were in a paradise where everything was planned for us, and we hardly had to think, but while the retreat was opulent and relaxing, I found myself eager to return to my regular life. This surprise made me reflect on the nature of purpose in our later years.

I imagine that many people want to retire to live the yoga retreat life, but for me, the retreat was wonderful *because* it was temporary. The time in Mexico felt purposeless to me. Easy, yes. Glamorous, certainly. But not how I want to spend all my time on earth.

As we age, the philosophy of shibui encourages us to embrace new challenges and continue growing rather than withdrawing from active engagement with life. It's about refining our purpose, not relinquishing it. What if we considered retirement to be a new segment of our evolution?

TANTANTO AND THE MIDDLE WAY

AS I'VE GROWN OLDER, I've found myself increasingly drawn to the Japanese concept of *tantanto*, a principle that aligns beautifully with the shibui approach to aging.

In my younger years, my brain compelled me to uphold an impossibly arduous work schedule. "More!" my psyche would growl as I mentally whiplashed about. Although I ascribed this tendency to my Japanese roots and work ethic, my parents were actually quite lax, cheerfully accepting that I might never reach great heights in my career.

"Tantanto, Sanae-chan. Tantanto," my mother would say when I pushed myself to exhaustion, mewling about burnout for the umpteenth time. The meaning of tantanto, like so many Japanese notions, is hard to elucidate in English. It's about going with the flow in a light, detached manner—a sort of laissez-faire attitude. It's the opposite of striving, but it's not giving up either. Perhaps the Buddhist tenet of the middle way comes pretty close in definition.

I hear my mother's voice in my head often: "Tantanto, Sanae-chan. Tantanto," those words replacing the demanding "More!"

Embracing tantanto as we age doesn't mean abandoning our goals or passions. Instead it's about donning a sense of ease and acceptance as we would a much-loved, imperfectly perfect handmade parka (one which I've sewn in a tantanto manner). Thus fortified and prepared for the elements, we trundle through life's ups and downs. It's recognizing that sometimes the most beautiful and meaningful moments come not from pushing harder but from allowing things to unfold naturally. If we can be at peace with circumstantial downpours, we'll also be treated to glorious, fleeting rainbows—every vacillation held temperately, tantanto.

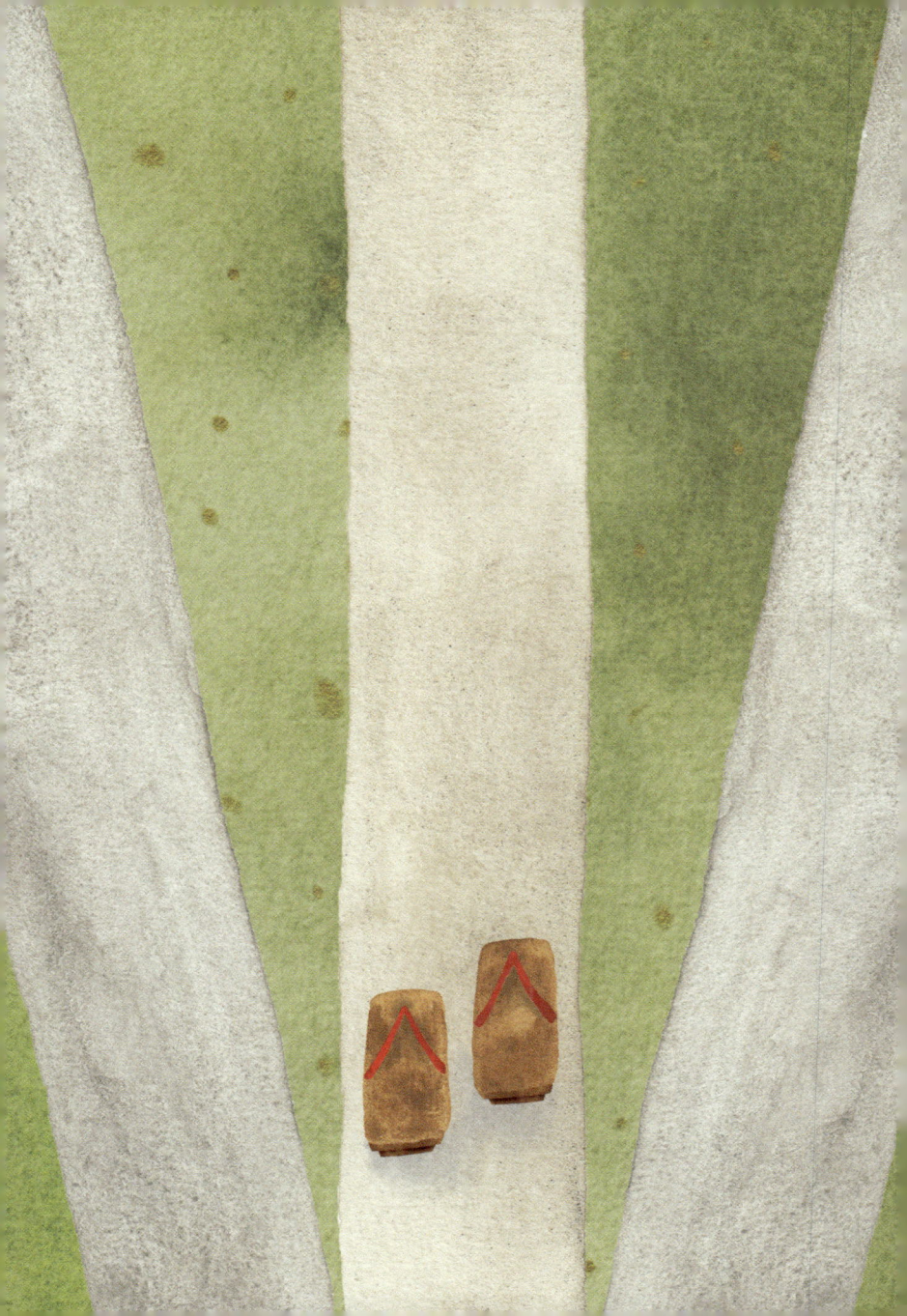

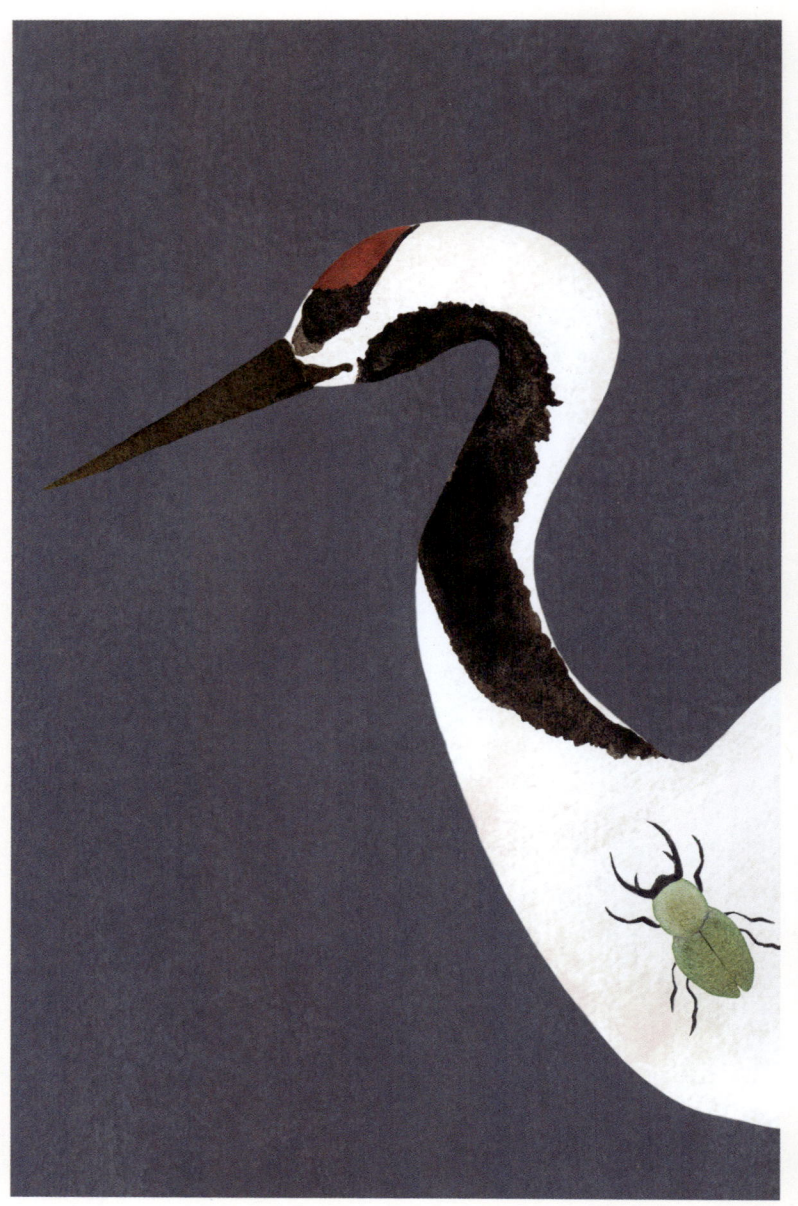

WHITE ENVY AND URAYAMASHII

OVER THE YEARS, MY view of envy has morphed signifi-
cantly. The green-eyed monster used to cause shame, but
no longer! The Russian concept of "white envy" (unlike
its counterpart "black envy") and the Japanese notion of
urayamashii offer insightful perspectives.

White envy connotes yearning for qualities we value
in others, accompanied by genuine appreciation that such
qualities exist. Urayamashii in Japanese culture is similar,
acknowledging admiration without bitterness. In Japan
I've noticed people express their urayamashii feelings
casually, often playfully.

I believe envy is one of the best indicators of our
truest desires. White envy guides us toward our purpose, providing clues to our existence. For years I was
simultaneously envious of and invigorated by writers
and illustrators. But once I allowed myself to create,
the envious feelings dissipated. What do you feel
urayamashii about?

Aging provides the opportunity to move from the
gnawing, covetous "black envy" of youth to an apprecia-
tive "white envy"—a refinement that enhances our beauty
as we age.

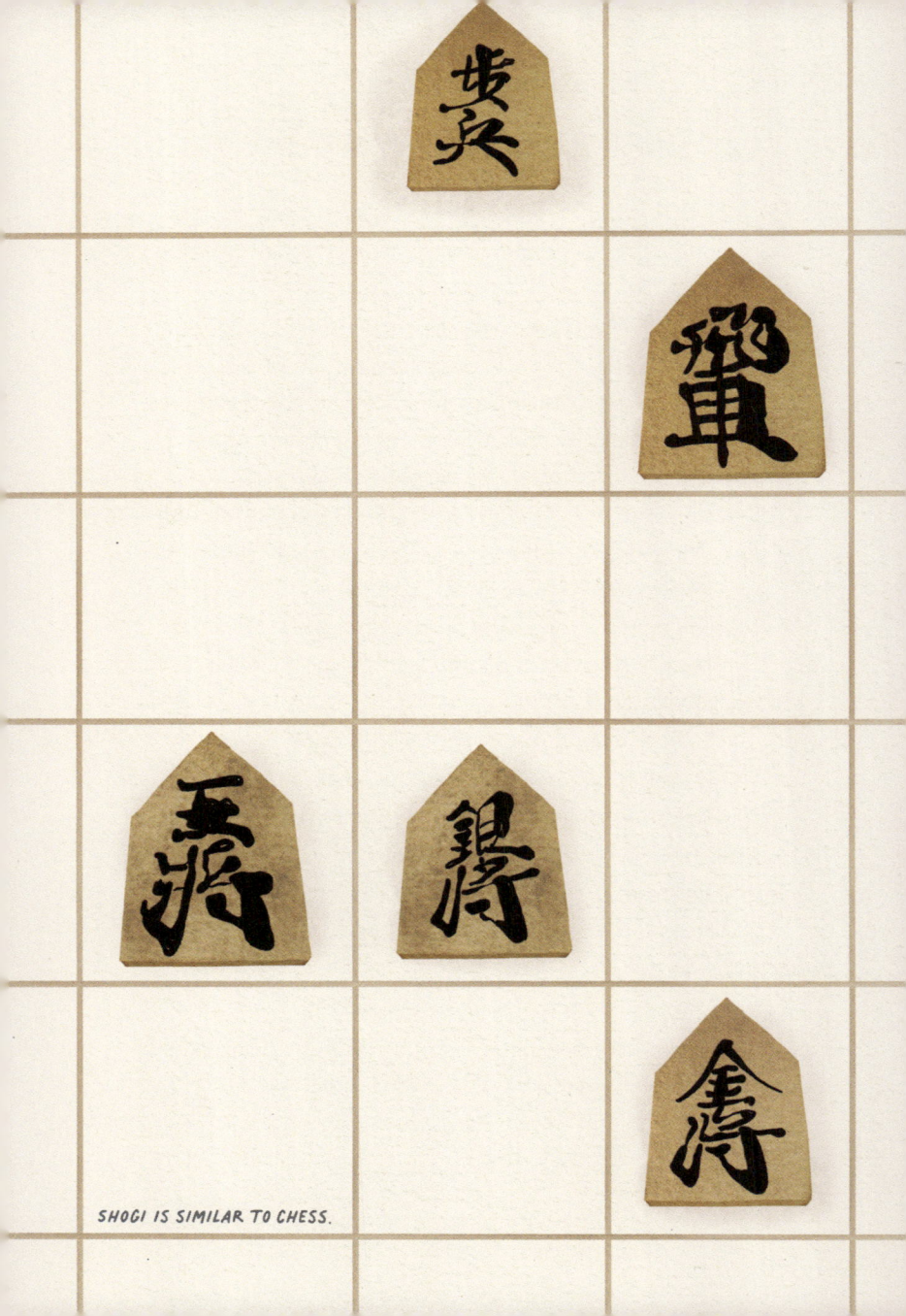

SHOGI IS SIMILAR TO CHESS.

SHIGOTO HARD, PLAY HARD

A NARROW, WINDING LANE hugs the curve of the small mountain in Shizuoka, Japan, where my parents reside. Even their miniature Nissan minivan—smaller than a compact car—barely fits on this road, and the slaloming trek up to their mountaintop village is both nauseating and breathtaking. On one side is the seascape with intriguing rock formations—one looks strikingly like a lion guarding the majestic waters. On the other side, there's dense, abundant forest as far as the eye can see.

Originally built as a collection of resort facilities in the 1990s, this tiny village has been transformed into a self-selected senior community. This seems an unlikely haven for seniors; there are no shops or medical facilities nearby, wild and poisonous animals roam the forests, and the houses perch precariously on hillsides with numerous stairs—yet the residents thrive.

Their days are filled with a variety of *shigoto*, or tasks. Many of them grow vegetables and nurture fruit trees. My mom's own garden bursts with cucumbers, melons, *mikan* (mandarins), *shiso* (a Japanese herb), and cherry blossoms. She picks ripe *kaki* (persimmons) from her neighbor's tree to dry them into *hoshigaki* by infusing the persimmons in plum wine or sake. Residents have created a bartering system, exchanging foodstuffs and household goods. Social activities such as ping-pong clubs and *mochi*-pounding parties keep their minds and bodies active.

Their lifestyle is a beautiful embodiment of the shibui approach to aging: prioritizing purposeful activity, communal connection, and the joy in everyday tasks. They help each other too. When my dad fell off the roof clearing the gutters, the community rallied around him, and it was clear he'd forged solid bonds even later in his life.

In many ways, the remoteness of the village, inconvenient though it may be, encourages interdependence and resourcefulness. Mountain living isn't for the faint of heart, and it gives these seniors renewed energy and purpose, challenging the notion that aging necessitates a retreat from active living.

Work-Related Japanese Phrases

It's no secret that Japanese people are known for hard work. Japanese workplaces also prize collaboration and cooperative involvement. Here are some uniquely Japanese terms and facets of Japanese work:

KOTSU-KOTSU means working diligently in small measures.

SALARIMAN is the Japanese version of the word "salary man," and it refers to the ubiquitous nine-to-five corporate employee. There is an expectation of salarimen to engage in after-work parties and to commit their entire lives to one company.

KARŌSHI means death from overwork, and it's a real thing. It takes the phrase "word of warning" to a new level.

RADIO TAISO refers to the gentle morning exercises that many Japanese companies require employees to participate in at the start of the day. When I lived in Japan, I walked by a group of construction workers doing radio taiso every morning. The exercises are low-impact enough for the elderly, and it's common for small groups of senior citizens to practice radio taiso in parks early in the morning.

Those who know when they have
enough are rich.

TAO TE CHING

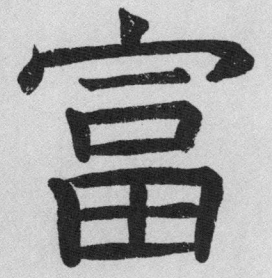

Tomi

WEALTH

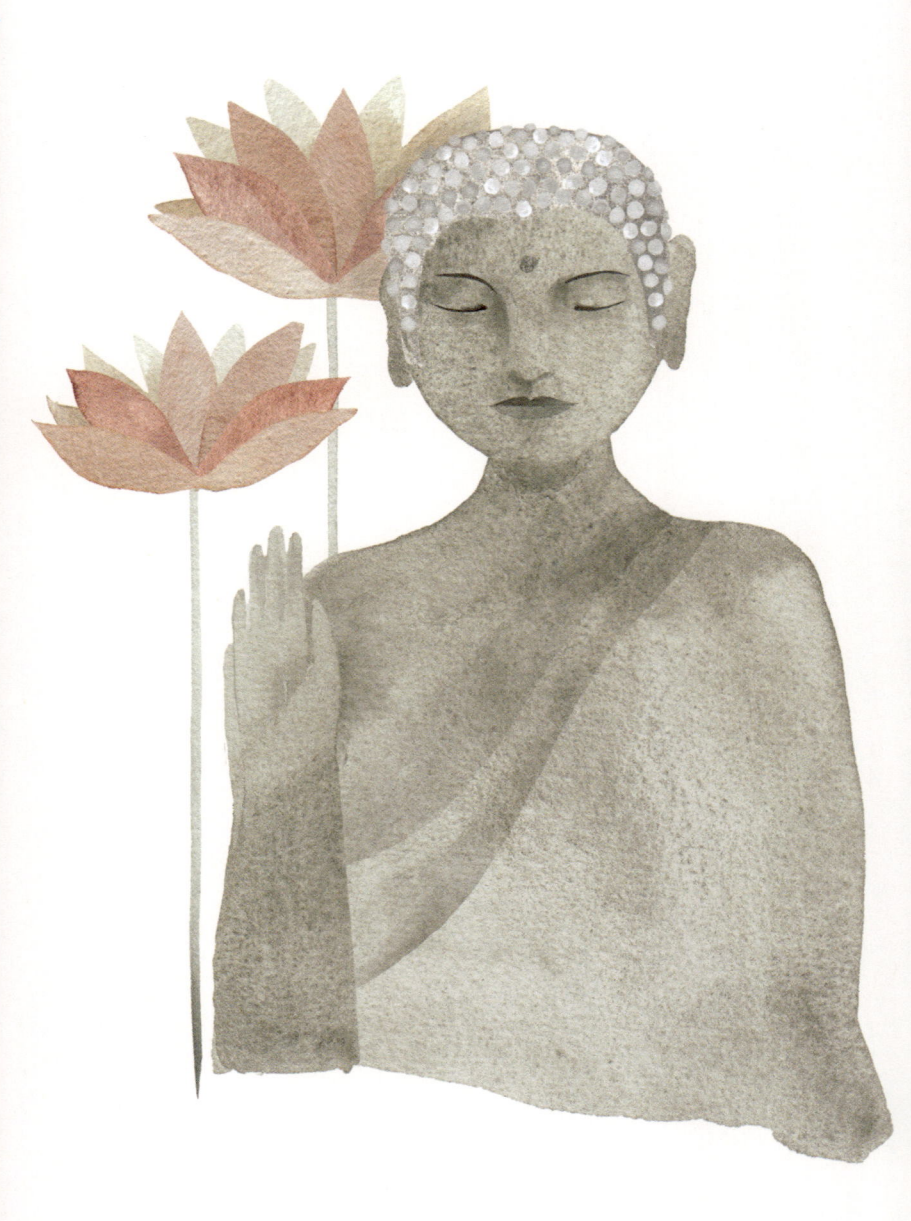

ON MEASURING WEALTH

THERE ARE SEVERAL WAYS to say "rich" in Japanese, just as the English language offers "wealthy," "affluent," and "prosperous." In Japanese, *tomi* translates directly to material wealth, but it also means general abundance. The exploration of true wealth is a perennial human conundrum. It's clearly more than material accumulation, yet we increasingly use money and status as primary measures.

As we age, our relationship with wealth transforms. What seemed valuable in youth—possessions, status symbols, external validation—gradually gives way to seeking and finding more ineffable richness. Shibui eschews glorification of gaudy displays, favoring simple elegance instead. There is a heartfelt gratitude for intangible wealth: the transitory beauty of seasons, the slow ritual of a tea ceremony, and other quiet celebrations of a well-lived life.

The shibui perspective recognizes the unexpected abundance that comes not from having more but from wanting less and appreciating what we already have. True wealth is measured by what we've come to value moments of connection, quiet contentment, and subtle joys often unnoticed in our earlier years.

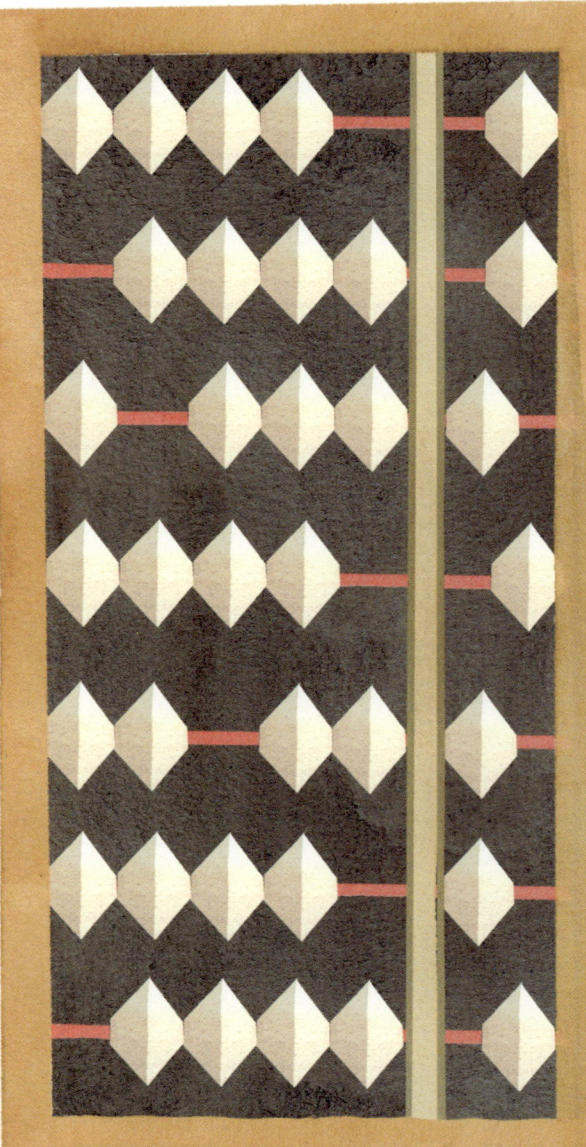

A VERY, VERY RICH LIFE

IT WAS IN A DIRTY, dusty, and mostly empty enclave in Lumbini, Nepal, where Prince Siddhartha Gautama—better known as Buddha—was purportedly born in 623 BCE. Immersed in their Buddhist era, my parents took my brothers and me there to stay in a plain, all-white monastery. It was 1983, and I was twelve years old.

On the day of our departure, a monk sat us all down on floor mats, side by side, for impromptu palm readings. First he gripped my mom's hand, leaned close, and stared at her palm for a few intense seconds. "Long life," he pronounced. Then he shuffled down the line on his knees, took hold of my eleven-year-old brother's hand, and studied his palm for even longer. "Fame!" he barked.

Shuffle, shuffle. The monk-cum-fortune teller maneuvered himself in front of my dad, turning his hand over and over as he peered at the etched lines. He gazed at my dad's face for an uncomfortable minute, and then, without saying a word, he made his way to me. The old monk's grip was firm, and his fingers felt cool. After a quick glance, he declared, "A very, very rich life." At twelve I couldn't possibly understand what richness truly meant.

Rich. The word conjures up images of towering piles of money, sleek and technologically advanced modes of transportation, sprawling manors, haute couture clothes, limitless luxury products, endless travel, entourages, and exclusive memberships to astronomically priced clubs. When I think of rich, I think of Beyoncé.

I have yet to experience the standard-issue accoutrements of wealth, and I don't know what Beyoncé's lifestyle actually looks like beyond the glamorous public image. My only point of reference is from my dad who was a chauffeur in Los Angeles—he gave her a lift once and thought she was very nice.

But now, at fifty-four, I look back on a life rich beyond belief. The best part of reaching this decade of my life is not only understanding but embodying what truly matters: love, freedom, well-being, and meaningful ways to occupy my days. None of these require vast sums of money, but they do demand the currency of awareness and acceptance that often becomes refined with age.

That dusty monastery in Nepal now seems fitting. Its unadorned architecture houses a trove of wisdom, much like a life that appears ordinary on the outside but contains immeasurable wealth within. Perhaps this is what the monk saw in my twelve-year-old palm: not material riches but a life that would grow richer with each passing year as I learned to value the quiet, meaningful moments that comprise a truly wealthy existence.

Ōbai tōri

Akin to the famous quote ascribed to Theodore Roosevelt that "comparison is the thief of joy," the Japanese idiom *Ōbai tōri* encourages celebrating unique strengths and bypassing comparison. Ōbai tōri is a conglomeration of four kanji letters that represent four trees that flower in the spring: cherry, plum, peach, and apricot. Each tree blooms in a distinct way at its own pace. No single tree type is better than the others, just as no individual person is better or more worthy than others. And all the blooms will eventually fade and fall away, as will our human bodies. Clearly the shibui philosophy that upholds the seasonality and beauty of nature is at play in Ōbai tōri.

Four kanji characters comprise Ōbai tōri: cherry blossom (桜, *sakura*), plum (梅, *ume*), peach (桃, *momo*), and apricot (李, *ri*).

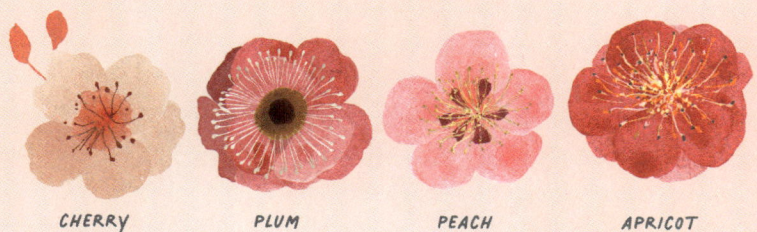

CHERRY   PLUM   PEACH   APRICOT

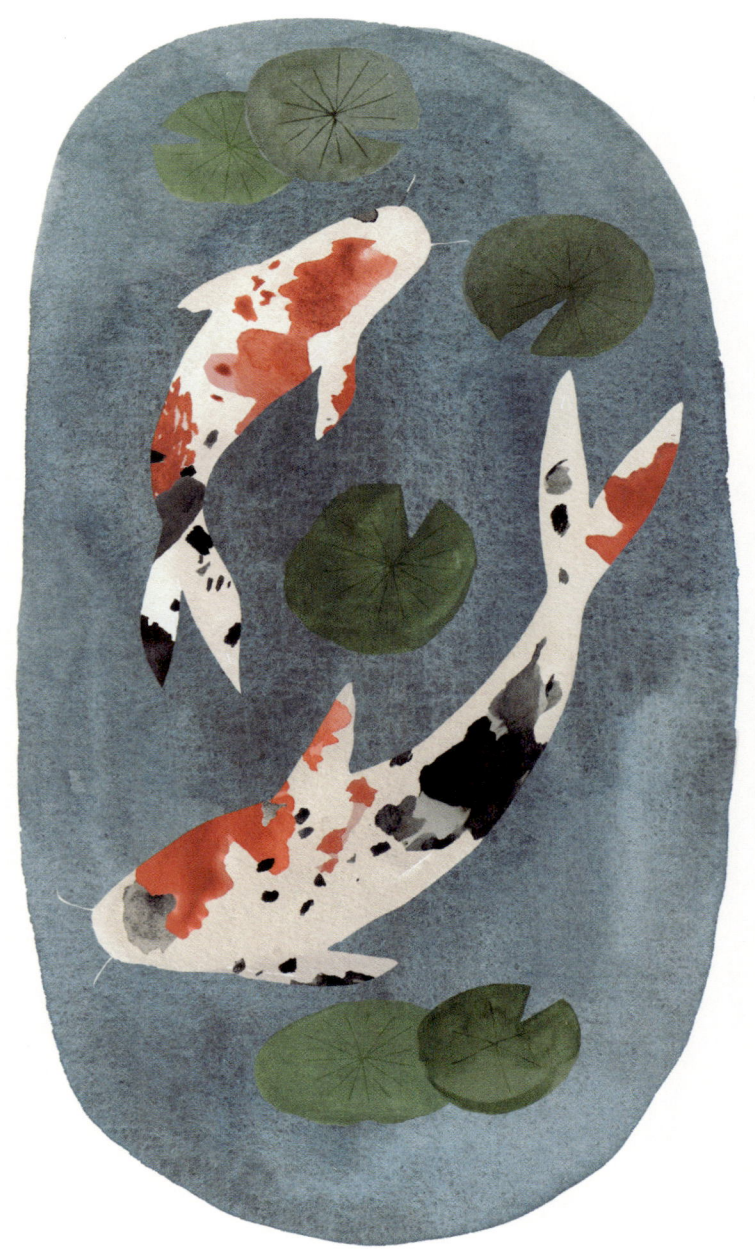

KEEPING UP WITH THE
JONESES AND SHIBUIS

IN MY TWENTIES, I got into debt. A lot of debt. My credit card balance ballooned with interest each month, and my school loan payments seemed interminable. I was mystified. I am a highly educated woman with a master's degree. I have been employed by Fortune 500 companies. According to the test administrator from second grade, my IQ score is above average. Yet as I stared at my credit card statements each month, I had to concede that something wasn't working quite right with my brain. For a supposedly smart person, I did (and still do) a lot of dumb things.

The story of how I got out of debt is a long, painful, and boring one. The reason for getting into debt in the first place is straightforward: I was intent on keeping up with the Joneses.

Online shopping and credit cards made this easy. When I was younger, my self-worth was entangled with external validation and comparison. Each purchase promised to fill a void, to make me feel as though I belonged.

Now, with the perspective that comes with age, I see how empty that pursuit was. On a recent visit to Japan,

I noticed that it is still a mostly cash-based society. And as I've learned from my parents, the Japanese are savers. If the Joneses are all about showing off things they don't really want, with money they really don't have, to impress people whose opinions don't matter, then perhaps the anti-Joneses are the shibui folks living authentic, connected lives within their means.

Shibui wealth is the opposite of flashy and gaudy. I've heard the term "quiet luxury" thrown about lately, and that veers closer to the Japanese concept. Shibui luxury isn't lavish. It's the lovingly handcrafted, plain bowl in which a simple but beautiful dish is served. Shibui is eating that dish slowly, savoring all the mingling flavors. It is an immersion in gratitude before, during, and after the experience. It's internal and not meant for flaunting. It is, in short, incomparable.

I've found liberation in this shibui approach to wealth over the years. There's a bolstering comfort in no longer measuring my worth against others' possessions or achievements. Instead I've learned to appreciate the subtle richness of what I already have—deepening relationships forged over decades, skills honed through years of practice, moments of inner beauty that require no price tag. This shift didn't happen overnight, but gradually, like a slow ripening that brings out the sweetest flavors.

Important Reminders

On the way to the airport for a recent trip to Japan, our car got sideswiped by a semi-truck. An ear-splitting, grating noise filled the interior of the car, and our vehicle swerved off the freeway. Entirely discombobulated, my husband pulled over onto the shoulder, and the semi-truck did the same. There, on the side of the rear passenger door, was an imprint of a huge wheel. It looked artistic, like a circular flourish of calligraphy.

We were so lucky. Once we determined that no one was hurt, we hastily exchanged phone numbers to send proper paperwork later and rushed to the airport.

There is a Japanese word, *mieppari*, that refers to a person hung up on maintaining appearances or caring too much about status and impressing others. My mom has always called me a mieppari, and younger Sanae would have been aghast to have that wheel imprint on the car. What would people think?"

Now that I'm older and nominally wiser, I find it symbolic: it represents the wabi-sabi aspect of shibui of finding beauty in imperfection. Why yes, I *do* find the wheel imprint quite fetching, and I haven't bothered to get it repaired. Life is precious. To be alive is a miracle. And hey, that circle looks rather like a shibui persimmon.

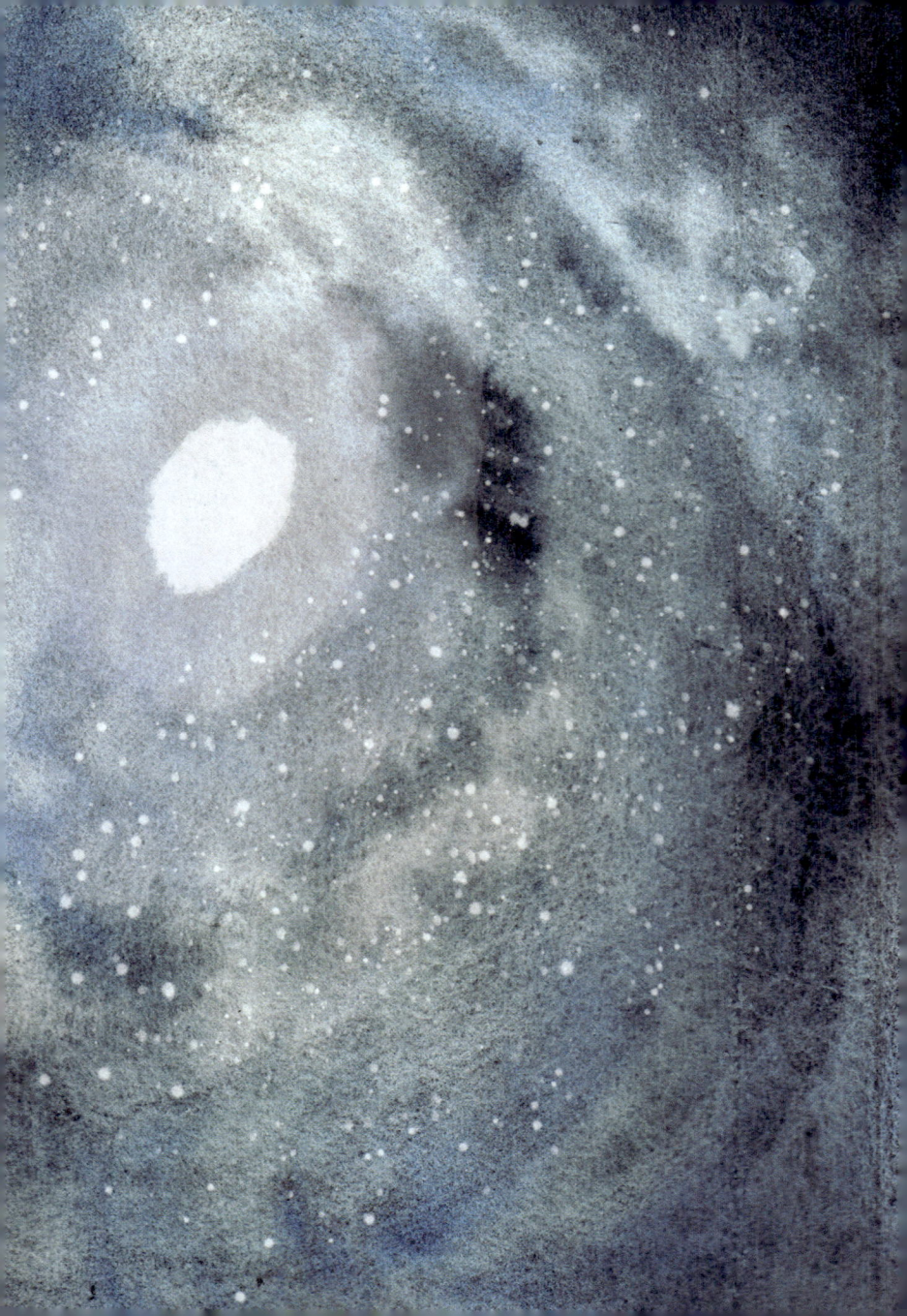

SUPPORTING ROLES

A FEW YEARS AGO, I was lounging in a coffee shop when I rose to get water. Something felt vaguely off, but I ignored it. In the bathroom a while later, I realized that my skirt had gotten tucked into my tights, exposing my bottom to the entire café.

Aging comes with the benefit of caring less and less about how ridiculous I may appear. This acceptance of my own imperfections is like a massive unshackling. Peace and freedom! It's as though I've been a falsely accused inmate for most of my life and have suddenly found the key to a spectacular jailbreak. The prosperity of placidity has increased with the years.

I've learned that, in general, no one pays much attention to me. And if they do, I'm just a momentary blip in their consciousness. I love the phrase, "We are all supporting roles in other people's mental movies." In Japanese these supporting roles are called *waki-yaku*, suggesting something peripheral, less important.

When my daughter was in high school, she spent hours on her hair and make-up, catastrophizing every pimple and each "trash hair day" or "horrible outfit." I'd remind her, "Some people may notice and even criticize, but it's never about you. You're just a temporary distraction from their own self-consciousness." Had she experienced my café mishap, she would have spiraled into despair. Ah, youth—I don't miss it.

The Japanese word for the starring role is *shuyaku*. We are all stars in our personal mental realms, but aren't we also waki-yaku in this great cosmic production? Aging has made me aware of my paradoxical position: important because I'm meant to offer what's uniquely mine, yet insignificant in the vastness of galaxies.

This dual perspective—being both essential and humble—is quintessentially shibui. It's knowing when to step forward and when to step back, when to speak and when to listen. With age comes the realization that there is richness in being the supporting character, in observing more and performing less. The beauty of waki-yaku lies in freedom from the pressure to always be exceptional, to always be noticed. Instead it invites us to find meaning in the quiet corners of life, in the subtle moments that often go unrecognized but ultimately form the foundation of a well-lived life.

In embracing our role as waki-yaku, we discover one of aging's greatest treasures: the freedom to simply be ourselves without apology or expectation. We are all enough, we are all meant to be here.

Yutaka and Yutori

While "*tomi*" directly translates to wealth, two other Japanese concepts offer multilayered perspectives on abundance.

YUTAKA describes a life of leisurely abundance, lacking in nothing—not just material possessions but fulfillment and contentment.

YUTORI, particularly shibui in nature, refers to the peace derived from intentional simplicity. It encompasses mental, emotional, and physical spaciousness that allows for relaxation, creativity, and self-integration. The antithesis of rushing and hustling.

One small change that has brought more yutori into my life is eliminating the phrase "I'm busy" when asked how I'm doing. This automatic response had become a reflexive habit, a badge of honor in our productivity-obsessed culture. Now I pause to reflect: *How am I actually doing?* Even when most people may not expect a considered answer, this moment creates space for a more meaningful connection.

As I age, I increasingly distance myself from hustle culture. The constant striving for more feels at odds with the shibui appreciation of the present.

Consider what automatic responses you might replace to cultivate more yutaka and yutori in your daily interactions.

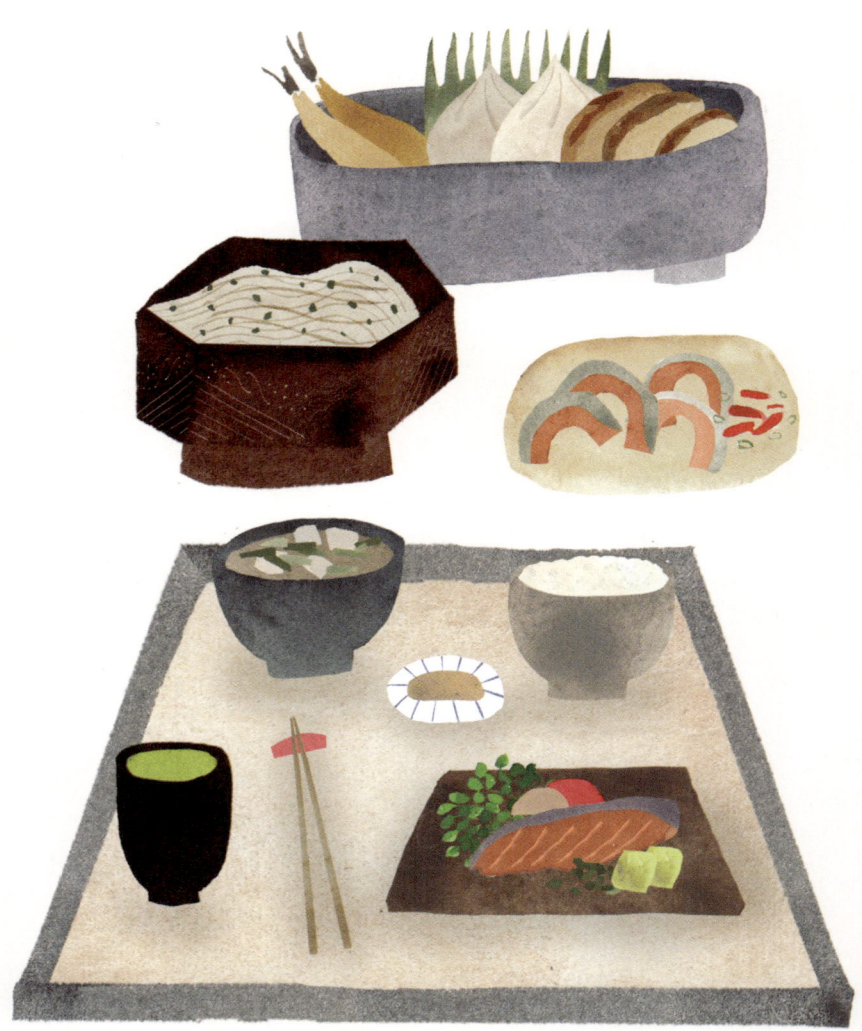

BOUNTIFUL LEFTOVERS

MY MOM IS A SUBLIME cook and has always made meals from scratch. No frozen pot pies or takeout for Okasan! My childhood was quite peripatetic, and the frequent relocations of my early years meant that I didn't really experience how other families lived. My parents shopped for groceries almost exclusively at Asian markets, so I thought that everyone else had fridges stuffed with odd-smelling, pickled, fishy, seaweed-y, and brown ingredients, and that rice was served with every meal.

Eventually, around third grade, I understood that we didn't have the money to spend on restaurant food, so meals usually consisted of whatever my mom could scrounge up from the pantry and refrigerator. As such I began to associate home cooking and leftovers with scarcity and shame. After I left home, I avoided cooking and subsisted on food from cheap eateries and sandwiches. I dabbled with cooking when I got married and gave birth, but processed and convenience foods dominated my diet.

Enter health crises. When I got sick in my forties, I overhauled my food intake, and ironically, I started cooking foods reminiscent of my mom's dishes. I realized

I had been turning up my nose at the wholesome, healthy foods my mom had served every day.

And the leftovers! Why did no one tell me that they make life so much easier, so much richer? When I come home famished from running errands in the morning, what a beautiful sight it is to behold the leftovers in my refrigerator. And they are even more wondrous on evenings when I'm too tired to cook, and the thought of going out is daunting. In a matter of minutes, I can heat up and nosh on a healthy, filling meal. It feels *decadent*. Luxurious. Now I get it.

This outlook on leftovers is equally apt for aging. What once seemed inadequate, embarrassing, or even undignified—leftovers, gray hair, laugh lines—can transform into something incalculably valuable. Just as a second-day stew often tastes better than the first serving, the flavors having been allowed to meld with layered umami, many aspects of life improve with time and patience.

Aging in a shibui way celebrates this kind of transformation—finding abundance where we once saw scarcity, recognizing wealth in what we already possess. My refrigerator full of leftovers has become a metaphor for the richness of my later years: a collection of experiences, relationships, and wisdom that sustains me in unexpected ways, providing nourishment that I undervalued in my youth.

WANTING WHAT I HAVE

I PEER INTO THE fifteen-times magnifying mirror, carefully applying shimmery taupe eyeshadow. I angle my face this way and that. *Nice*, I think, then toss the eyeshadow palette into a drawer with at least a dozen other similar ones.

As my face shows more signs of aging, I seem to collect more products designed to enhance or conceal these changes. I continue hunting for the elusive, perfect shimmery taupe shadow. Whenever I see a new brand or formulation, a greedy monster within me rises, shouting, "Get it get it get it! This one might be *the one!*"

I do the same thing with watercolor paints and skincare products. Something inside convinces me that better is always out there, not yet in my possession. Despite escaping my debt-ridden past, this insatiable voice persists. I'm careful not to overspend now, but the urge remains.

Clearly it's not the eyeshadow or moisturizer that I truly want, but the idea of beauty that advertisers peddle. The watercolor paints won't magically bestow the skills I admire in others. In short, I avoid using what I already have—when I have so much. It's something I'm more aware of as I get older, and I lean more into minimalism. The search for external validation is time-consuming and space-filling. Instead I reach toward the shibui philosophy of appreciating what is already present, finding beauty in what others might overlook.

This quest to fill inner voids with material goods or external validation often leads to debt, hoarding, and diminished self-esteem. When caught in this trap, I think of my friend's daughter, Lily, when she was three years old. Gazing into a mirror, she declared, "I'm amazing!" Yes, she is amazing. We're all amazing exactly as we are and become even more so with age. I'm slowly reclaiming this childlike self-acceptance, now enriched by the depth of experience.

I love Arthur Ashe's wisdom:

Start where you are.
Use what you have.
Do what you can.

And I would add, *Want what you have.*

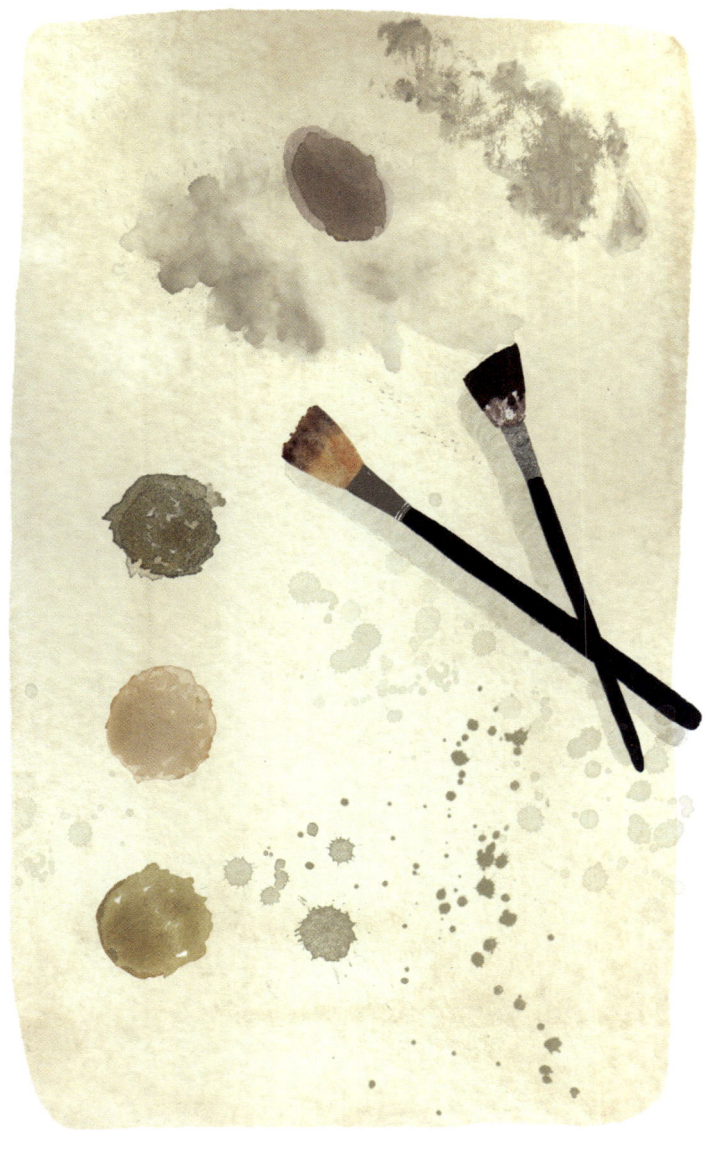

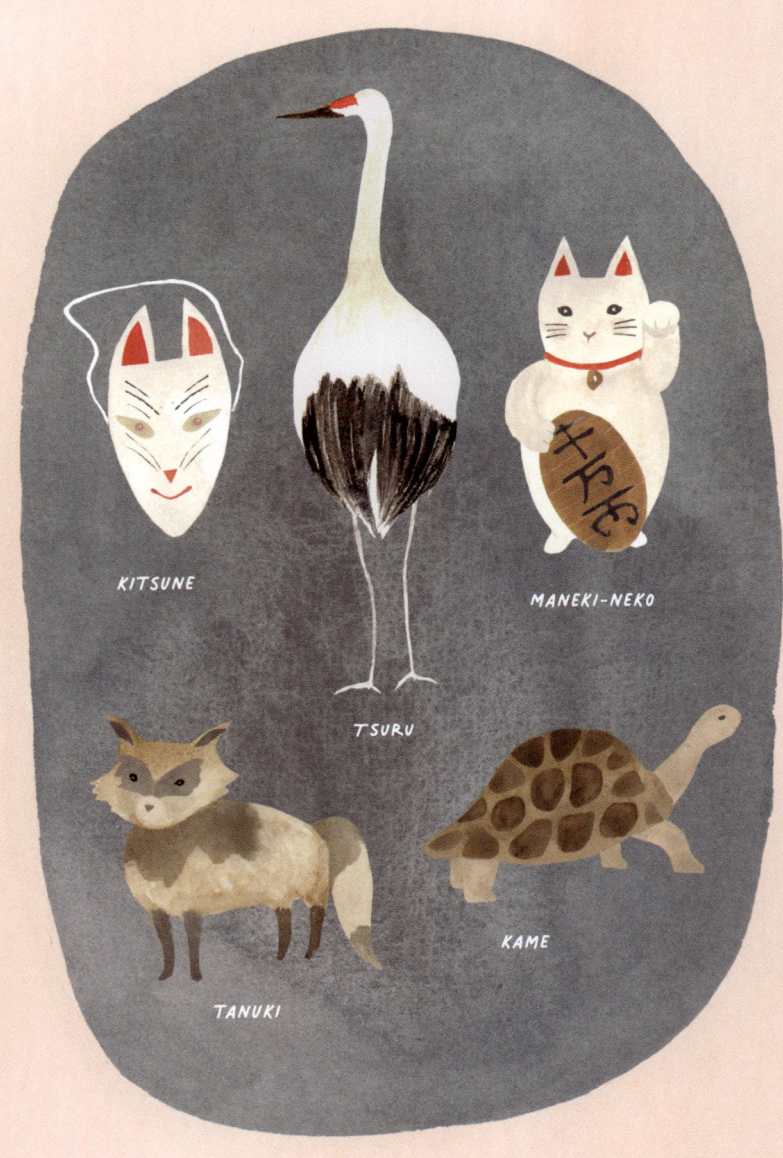

KITSUNE

TSURU

MANEKI-NEKO

TANUKI

KAME

Symbols of Wealth in Japan

In Japanese culture, wealth and good fortune are represented through various symbols that aligns with the shibui principles of subtle beauty and depth. Many are ubiquitous and part of every imaginable aspect of Japanese life, including comic book elements, train station ads, and home goods.

MANEKI-NEKO: This beckoning cat is associated with prosperity. Small ceramic maneki-nekos are placed at the entrance of many shops to invite abundance.

KITSUNE: Long associated with the rice spirit, the cunning fox symbolizes good fortune and is often found at Inari shrines (devoted to the god Inari), growing more revered with age.

TANUKI: The Japanese raccoon dog is ascribed a mischievous, rascally personality but can be a propitious bearer, often depicted with a round belly symbolizing contentment.

TSURU: In Japanese art, cranes are symbols of longevity, auspiciousness, wisdom, peace, and loyalty.

KAME: Because of the turtles' naturally long lifespans, they represent longevity, *chie* (wisdom), and positive luck—a living embodiment of the beauty of aging.

*Life is a balance between holding
on and letting go*

RUMI

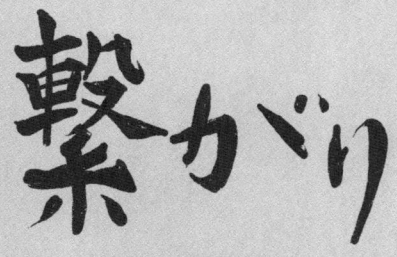

Tsunagari

CONNECTION

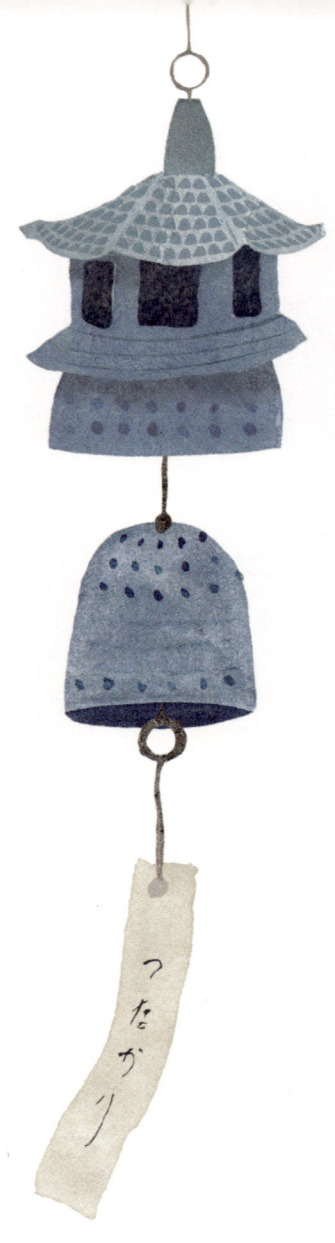

つながり

JAPANESE WIND CHIMES CALLED FŪRIN SYMBOLIZE INTERCONNECTEDNESS.

ON CONNECTING

I ATTENDED FIVE ELEMENTARY schools across Los Angeles and had a short second-grade stint in Tokyo. I learned how to make friends quickly but also to let go of them just as rapidly.

My mother has apologized for the constant uprooting—my parents were doing their level best as immigrants with limited resources. The apology surprised me. Though it wasn't an easy childhood, it endowed me with a noteworthy skill: adaptability.

This adaptability is a cornerstone of shibui living, which involves an all-encompassing acceptance and willingness to shift, pivot, learn, and connect. I use it to navigate my marriage, my friendships, my family relations, and my work environments. While our society emphasizes permanence and stability, the shibui perspective honors the beauty in transformation, respects seasonal intransience, and cherishes all types of interconnections.

With age comes a deeper understanding of *tsunagari*—the Japanese expression for connection—not as something to be clenched but as an ever-evolving web of relationships that shape us. The beauty is in the graceful dance of holding on and letting go.

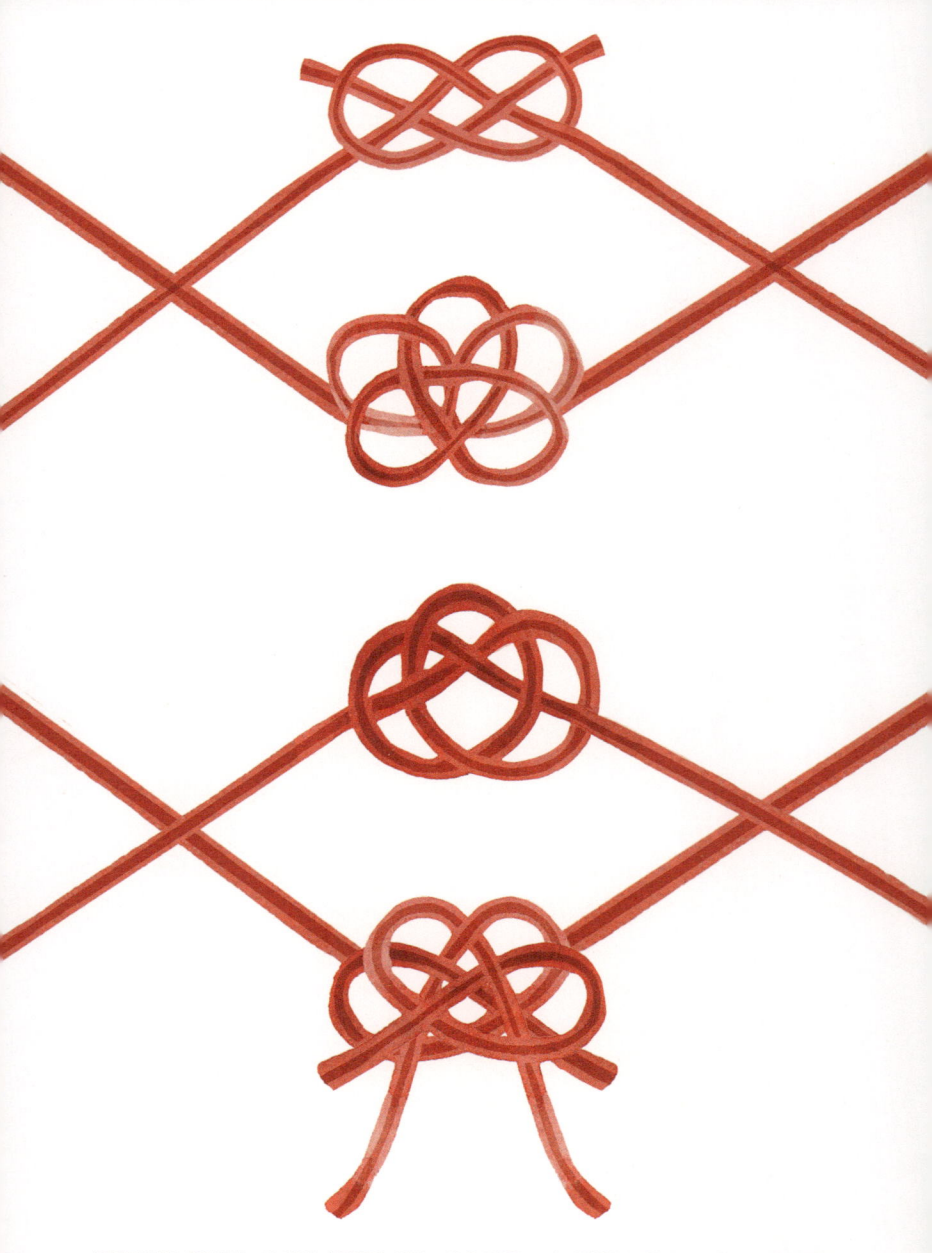

MIZUHIKI KNOTS ADORN GIFTS AND ARE USED AS CELEBRATORY DECORATIONS.

WIZENED AND INTERTWINED

IN MY LATE TWENTIES, scrambling to find my calling, I sublet my San Francisco apartment to a friend for the summer, moved back in with my unamused parents, and joined a temp agency. I sought a change of pace, away from the Bay Area hamster wheel of success-chasing. After scoring a gig with a local nonprofit, I discovered a showbiz culture lacking the altruistic environment I'd imagined. This was Hollywood in the 1990s, after all.

Disillusioned, I ate lunch by myself and journaled every day. I remember staring blankly at the sidewalk during one particular lunch break. In my periphery, I saw a pair of tightly clasped hands. The hands were wizened, with a maze of faintly blue-green veins, an Andromeda of tiny light brown spots, knobby knuckles and joints, and an ethereal translucence to the skin. Had these hands held each other for decades? There was such an ease and familiarity.

Tears welled up, surprising me. I ached to know how they did it. *How can I be like you?* I wondered. *Will I find someone who will want to hold my hand when I'm shriveled and forgetful?*

My typical Japanese parents never touched, and had I seen them kiss, I might have gone catatonic with shock.

They stopped hugging me when I was about six or seven, and though I still embrace my mom from time to time, it's unthinkable to do so with my dad.

Touch, as we know, is vital to well-being. Its importance extends far beyond romance. I admire Western culture's comfort with exhibiting affection, and how it seems so open, so free when I contrast it with my bowing, reserved Japanese relatives.

That glimpse of intertwined, elderly hands still creates a yearning in me all these years later, but one bolstered by delicious anticipation. Maybe I found my calling that summer, after all—to give and receive love into old age.

There's a photo album I made for my husband nearly a quarter of a century ago when we first started dating and had traveled to Montana. I remember sprawling out on the ground by the river to soak in the big, big sky. He said to me, "This is exactly how I want us to be when we're fifty, fat, and gray—lying on the grass and enjoying ourselves."

Now that my husband and I are empty nesters, the days are quieter. After dinner he reaches across the table to hold my hand. We clasp fingers, and I notice that the skin on our hands is gradually, almost imperceptibly, changing. Our skin looks rougher, a tad mottled, less taut. Connections are meant to ebb and flow through the years, but our tsunagari has extensive, interlinking roots. Our marriage is unassuming, weathered, and beautifully shibui in its everydayness. Here we are, fifty-plus, gray, and easeful in our skins, wizened and intertwined.

Love and Its Many Forms

The word for love in Japanese is *ai*, though one could also use *suki*, which is a more lighthearted form of love equivalent to "like." *Daisuki* or "big like" can mean love too. As we age, our experience and expression of love become more nuanced and multifaceted—much like the Japanese language's approach to this emotion.

While the English-speaking world considers the heart and mind to be anatomically separate, the word for heart in Japanese is *kokoro*, but it has a broader meaning that represents the joining of the heart and mind as inseparable entities. The kanji character for kokoro is part of the word "ai," suggesting that true love engages both emotional and intellectual aspects of our being.

Japanese culture recognizes that our inner landscape can be either *semai* (narrow or constricted) or *hiroi* (spacious and expansive). As we age through a shibui lens, our kokoro ideally becomes more hiroi, able to encompass a wider range of experiences and emotions with equanimity.

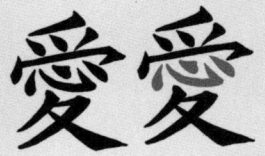

KANJI FOR LOVE (AI)
THE PORTION IN ORANGE IS THE
KANJI FOR HEART (KOKORO).

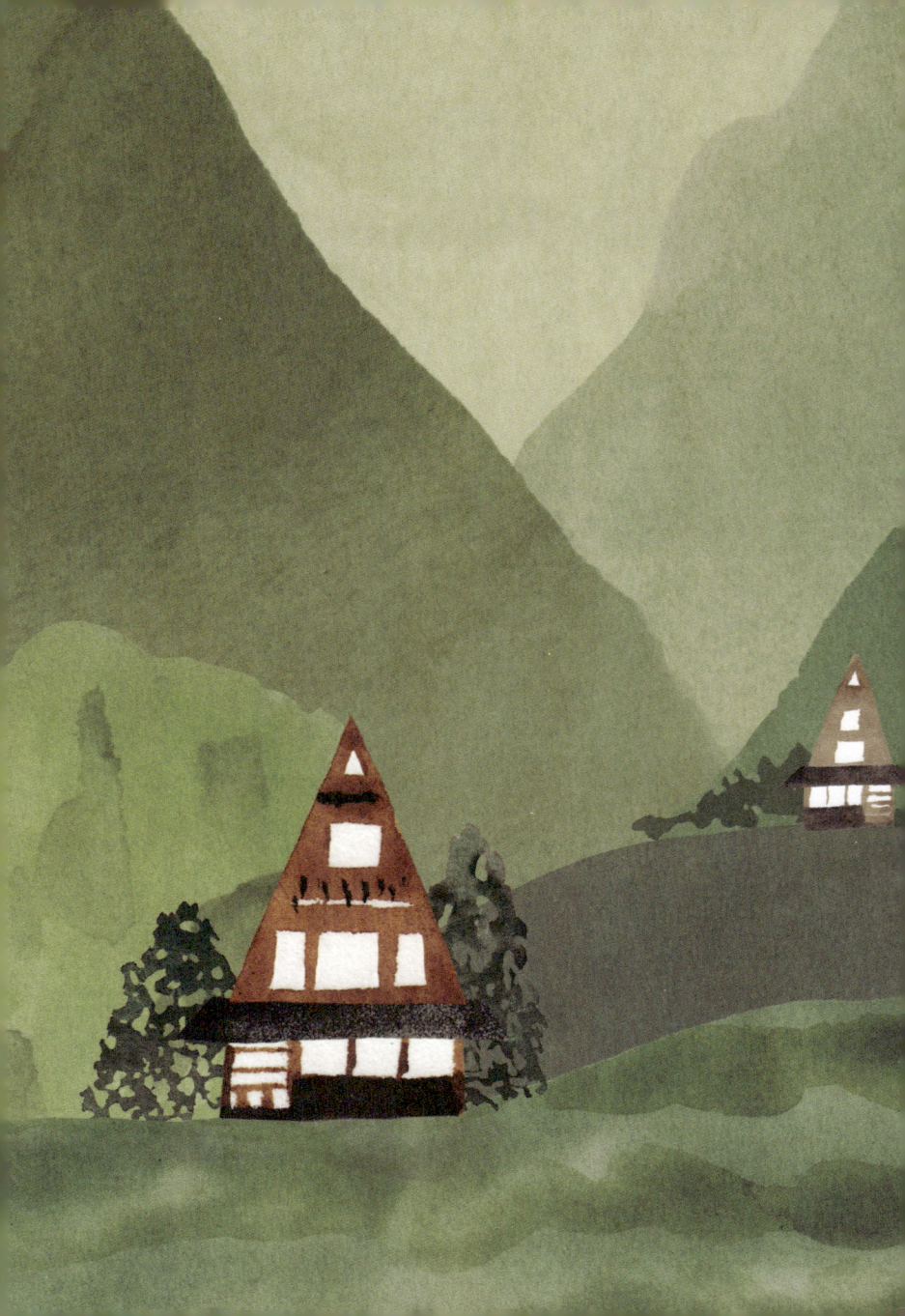

LOST

SPRING 1997. MIE PREFECTURE, Japan. I was a high
school English teacher in a small city through the Japan
Exchange and Teaching (JET) Programme and my friend,
a fellow JET instructor, asked me to help her scout
a potential campsite for a group trip. Due to a slight
schedule conflict, we agreed to take separate trains and
settled on a meeting place near the campsite.

When I made it to the base of the mountain, I
discovered that the bus to the campsite had stopped
running. *No problem*, I thought, *I'll hoof it*. So up the
mountain I went. Up and up and up. The trees grew
denser. The path narrower. Just as I was about to give
up, I came upon a vista reminiscent of the Japanese
folktales I had devoured as a kid. Little thatched-roofed
huts dotted wide fields. Tufts of smoke floated from the
chimneys. It was eerily quiet.

In front of one of the huts, an old woman in traditional Japanese work clothes crouched with a bowl and
wooden pestle.

"Excuse me!" I called out in Japanese. "Can you tell me
where the campsite is?"

She paused and stared at me. Then she rattled off a reply in a dialect so heavy that I didn't understand a word. She waved her arms toward the path.

Uncertain, I bowed in thanks and continued hiking. As the sky darkened, I halted. Where was I? How did I get off the main path? *Wait, is that an illustration of a bear on that sign?* Strange sounds emanated from the underbrush.

A distant drone grew louder, and then behind me, a tiny vehicle putt-putted onto the narrow path.

"You!" a voice yelled from the car as it screeched to a stop. "Are you the one looking for a campsite?" I nodded at a middle-aged woman, who sighed with relief and beckoned me into the car. The old woman in front of the hut was her mother who, fearing for my safety, had sent her daughter to find me. I nearly wept with gratitude.

The daughter took me to the campsite, but my friend was gone. She then drove me to the train station. Decades later I'm still touched by the incident. Despite the language barrier, the old woman intuited my plight and extended benevolence through her family. It was a brief encounter, yet I felt like I was part of a global tribe that always looks out for each other.

As I've grown older, these moments of unexpected care feel even more dear. They reveal a universal human connection that often strengthens with age—a willingness to reach out to strangers, to create tsunagari where none existed before. In the twilight of our lives, perhaps these simple acts of kindness become our most valuable exchanges.

UNIVERSAL INTERCONNECTEDNESS: SERENDIPITY

RECENTLY I PLANNED AN elaborate trip for my daughter and mom to explore Kyoto, Osaka, and Nara. On the second day of our Kyoto stay, I received an excited text from my friend saying that she'd just seen my daughter. She was on a bus and called out from the window, but we didn't hear her. I knew that my friend would be in Kyoto around the same time, but we weren't sure if we'd be able to meet up since she was with an organized tour group. What were the chances of this surprise encounter?

These types of coincidences happen all the time, yet they never cease to amaze me even as I grow older and discern how commonplace they are. My favorite synchronicity story also happened in Kyoto to someone I knew many years ago. We'll call him Max.

Max was traveling by himself. One day his growling stomach led him to wander the alleyways of Kyoto looking for a non-touristy restaurant. He found an unobtrusive pint-sized eatery and ducked in. Because it was in a less trafficked area, the restaurant employees didn't speak much English, and the menu was entirely in Japanese (Max neither spoke nor read Japanese).

It was Max's lucky day because the restaurateur's family friend who understood English happened to be upstairs. The young woman came down to translate the menu, and after he ordered, the two got talking.

"I am going to America soon," the young woman shared.

"Oh, that's where I live!" Max replied.

"How wonderful! Do you know Seattle, Washington? That is where I am staying," the young woman added.

"Amazing! I live in Seattle," Max exclaimed.

"I am staying with a friend's sister. I have not met her yet. I am so excited for my trip!"

And then it dawned on Max. This young woman he'd randomly met in a hole-in-the-wall restaurant in Kyoto was, in fact, going to be staying in *his* house in Seattle. The friend's sister was his wife!

In terms of coincidences, that one's hard to beat. And it reinforces something that we all intrinsically understand: we are all interconnected.

Interconnectedness is a core aspect of shibui, and as we traverse the timeline of our lives, these unexpected, invisibly interwoven serendipities start to seem ordinary and inevitable, potentially part of an overarching synchronous design. They hold us all together as though we're nestled in a giant, galaxy-sized cocoon. Could it be that these are wise indicators of providence? "Take heed!" they may be encouraging. "Aging is not an end but a way to burst forth in magnificent, interdependent metamorphosis."

The Okinawan Lifestyle

The southernmost prefecture, located roughly four hundred miles from the mainland, Okinawa is part of the Blue Zone regions where people enjoy longer, healthier lives.

FOOD: Okinawans consume 70 percent less sugar than the average Japanese person. Their diets feature foods high in antioxidants, such as sweet potatoes and *gōya* (bitter melon). This bitter flavor—shibui in the gastronomical sense—is believed to contribute to longevity. The mineral-rich salt has also been gaining popularity as a healthy condiment.

ACTIVITY: Most Okinawans remain physically active into old age, practicing mokuteki (maintaining purpose and meaningful daily activity). With less furniture in their homes, they naturally strengthen mobility and muscles through regular squatting.

COMMUNITY: Aging is communal in Okinawa. Elders are respected and integrated into daily life. Multiple generations often live together, creating built-in family support. The traditional *moai* (social support groups formed in childhood) provide emotional, social, and even financial support throughout life.

SPIRITUALITY: Everywhere you turn in Okinawa, statues of lion-dragons called *shisa* stand guard. With roots hailing back to when trade started with China via the Silk Road, the shisa have been an integral, protective presence in Okinawa.

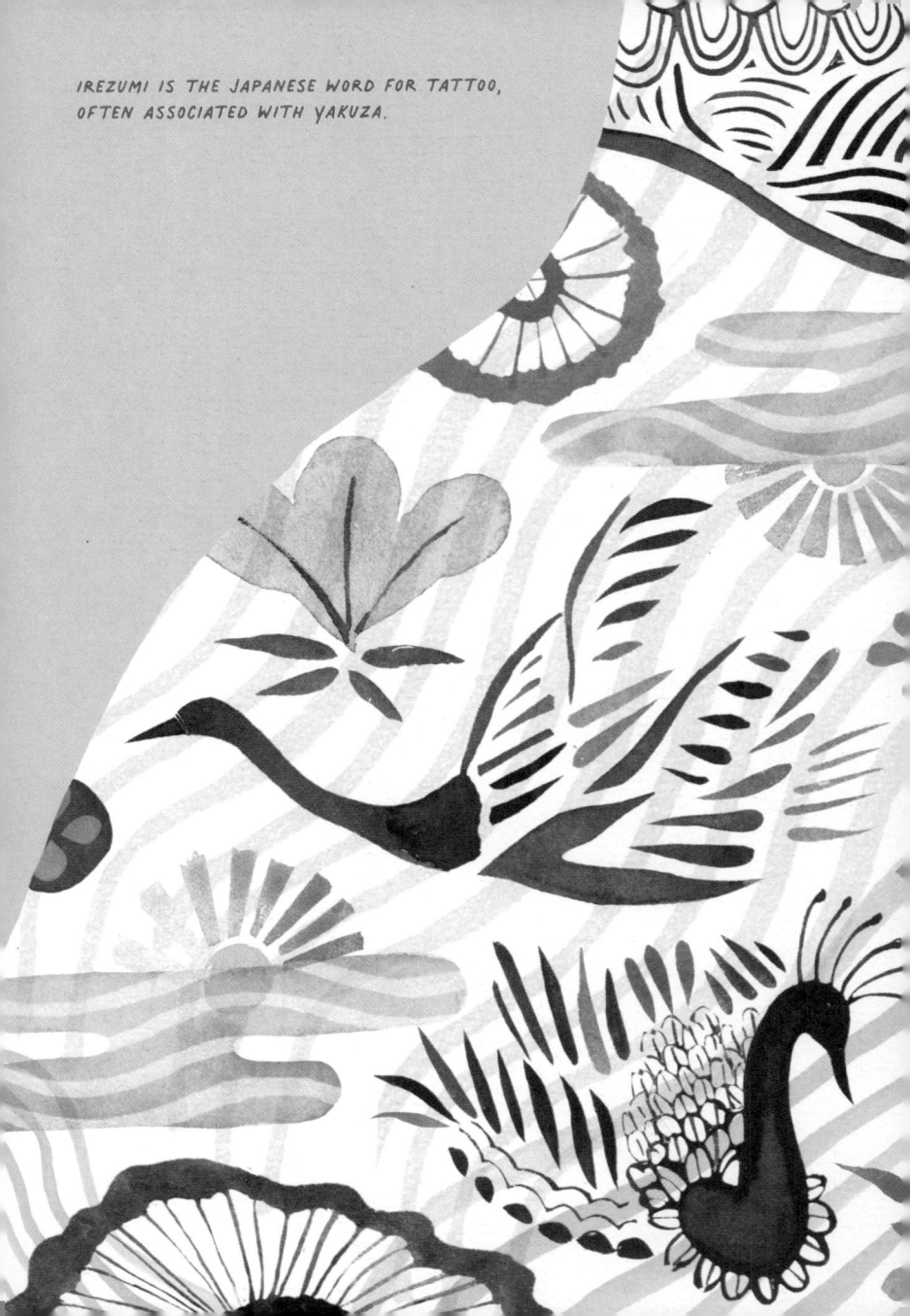

IREZUMI IS THE JAPANESE WORD FOR TATTOO,
OFTEN ASSOCIATED WITH YAKUZA.

EVEN THE YAKUZA RESPECT THE ELDERLY

WHEN I WAS TEACHING in Japan, my mom came to visit me and told me a funny story. She was struggling with her luggage at the train platform when a group of tough-looking youths approached her. My mom thought that they might be part of a Yakuza gang, and her guard went up. To her surprise, however, the youth politely offered to help her with the luggage. With swagger and a lot of noise, the boys carted her suitcase up the steps, then kowtowed with reverential bows and headed in the other direction. Delightful!

As we age in Western societies, we often become more invisible. This small incident reveals the Japanese culture's ingrained respect for the elderly that transcends social boundaries. Even those who might operate outside conventional norms still uphold certain cultural values. It's a respect that isn't merely performative; it's woven into the fabric of society.

As such, in the shibui perspective, aging isn't something to conceal or overcome, but rather a natural progression that confers a certain dignity and worth.

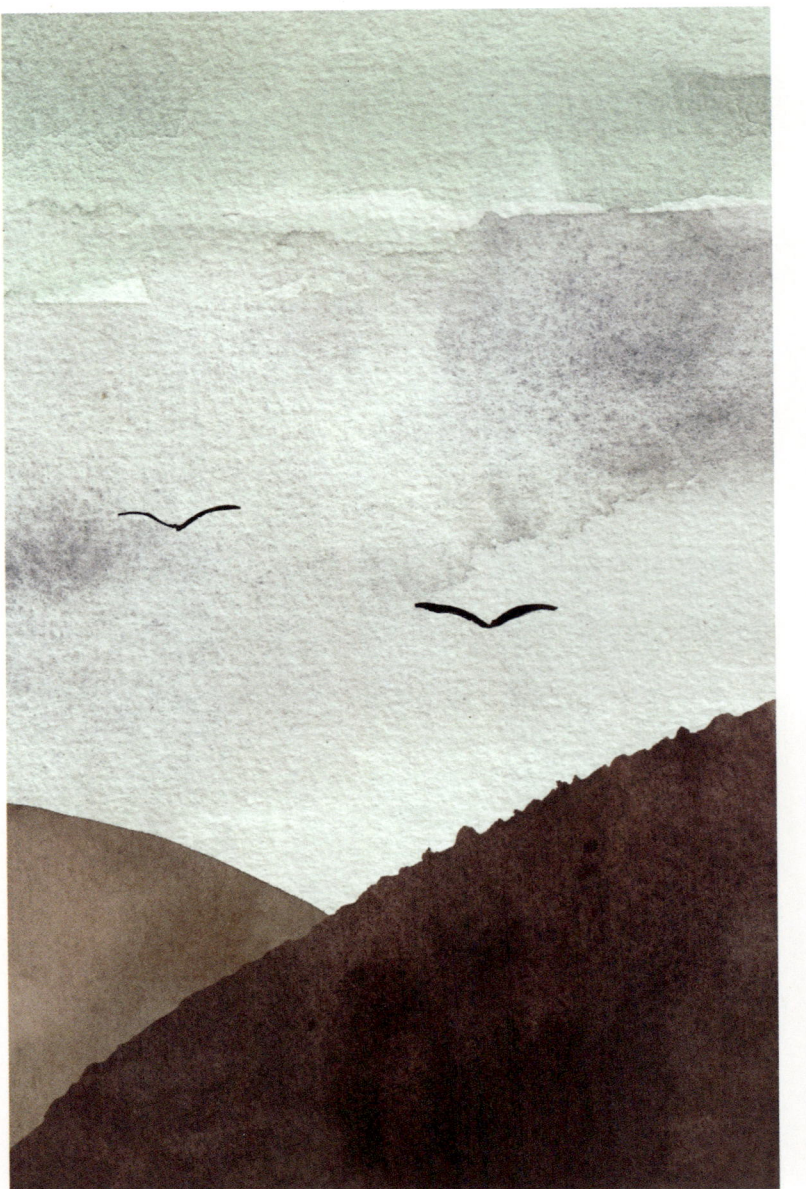

THE LONELINESS DIS-EASE

A COUPLE OF YEARS ago, I met a very famous celebrity at an author event where he was the keynote speaker. I mustered my courage to approach his signing table and, after a short wait, I handed him his book for a signature. When he saw my author name tag, he asked about my work. I stammered, blushed, and fidgeted, feeling utterly inadequate before this internationally recognized actor and comedian.

He leaned back, lacing his fingers to cradle the back of his head, and appeared ready for a lengthy conversation. Although there was no one waiting behind me, my sense of inferiority—though not as heightened as it had been in my younger years—drove me to flee after just five minutes.

I have thought about that event a lot. As humans, we naturally compare and stratify. I had created this imaginary hierarchy between us and ended up missing an opportunity to interact with an interesting person.

Shibui philosophy counters this tendency by teaching that we're all part of the universe—beautiful and flawed. Creating hierarchies contradicts this understanding of inherent beauty in everything, regardless of perceived status. Roses, for example, don't compare themselves to dandelions, as far as we know.

Age has helped me shed these artificial comparisons, and I value genuine connection over performative competition. Yet in my encounter with the celebrity, I reverted to adolescent insecurity—a reminder that aging doesn't automatically guarantee wisdom; we must continually practice it.

Today, despite greater digital connectivity, people construct unhelpful hierarchies that divide us. Loneliness has become an epidemic in this century. Our online sharing of "haves" and "have-nots" only magnifies this isolation.

We claim to seek authenticity while questioning our own identity. Perhaps one of aging's greatest gifts is this gradual removal of pretense, the quiet unfurling of our true selves from beneath the social masks we're wearing.

As Brené Brown wisely advises in her book *Atlas of the Heart*: "Don't shrink, don't puff up. Hold your sacred ground."

Kansha

Kansha means gratitude and thanksgiving, which are key elements of a well-aged, connected life. As we grow older, this practice of appreciation is like a centrifugal force for creating abundance and meaning in our human existence. It's difficult to feel deprivation when gratitude is at the core.

Japanese kanji are derived from Chinese characters and are pictographs—simplified visual representations of words and concepts. I love the kanji characters that comprise the word kansha, 感謝

It is made up of two characters:

感:The first character, kan, represents open-heartedness with the kanji 心 (heart) combined with 咸 (mouth, open).

謝:The second character, sha, combines 言 (words) and 身 (body) and 寸 (a Japanese measurement) and represents expressing gratitude.

This visual representation reminds us that true gratitude involves both feeling (heart) and expression (body and words)—a whole-person experience that deepens with age and practice.

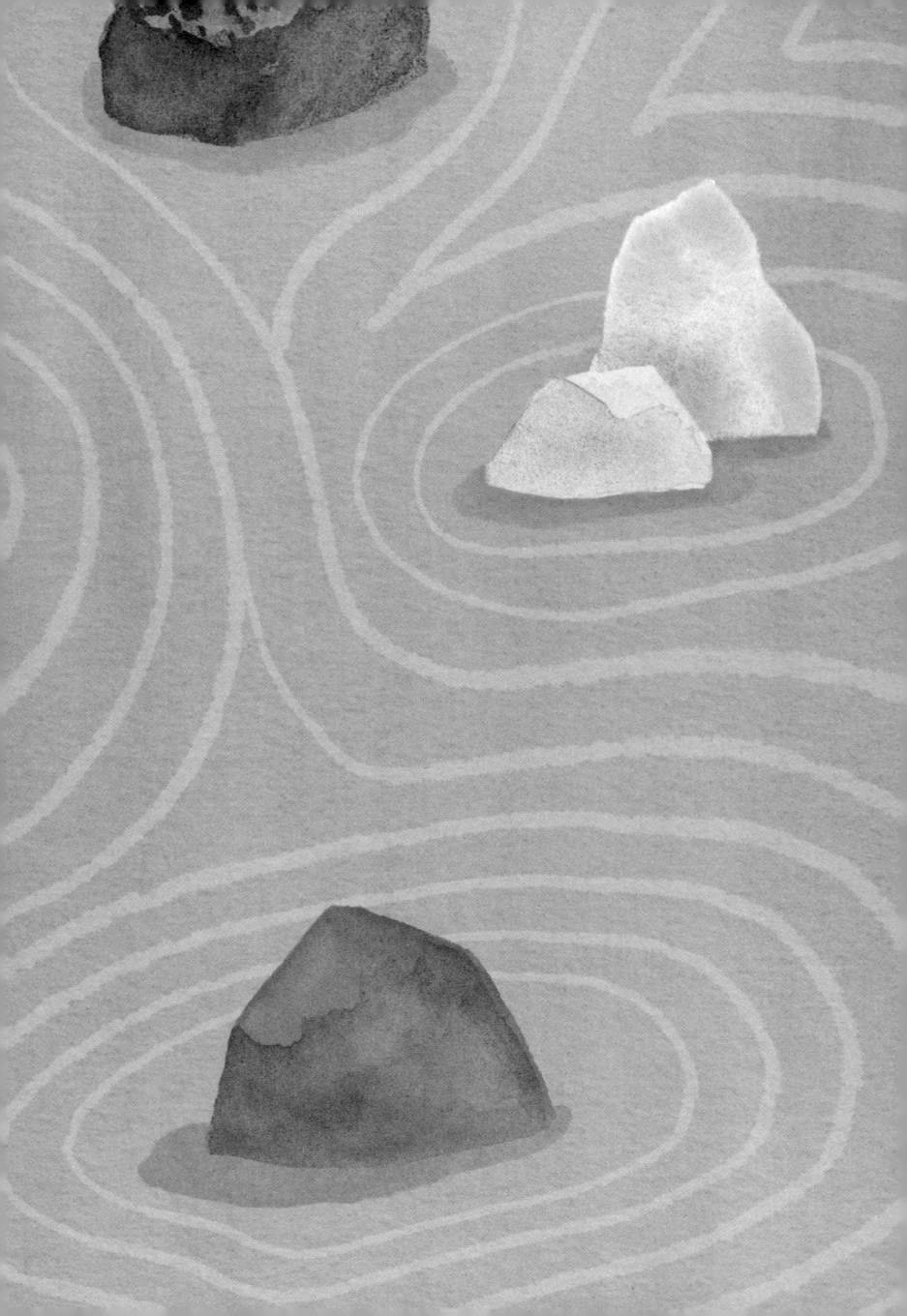

CARLESS IN SEATTLE

WHEN OUR OLD HONDA Civic finally died, something compelled me to hold off on replacing it. I'd lived without a car in Japan and San Francisco, and for the first four years in Seattle, my husband and I remained carless until our daughter came along. *We can do this!* I thought. I've always hated driving anyway.

It was difficult at first. Food shopping required extensive planning, and coordinating school activities and social events involved asking for many carpooling favors. My daughter felt embarrassed that we were different from other car-possessing families. My husband complained vociferously about the inconvenience.

Yet.

I walked for miles every day and became fit. I also felt calmer because I was practicing a kind of urban *shinrin-yoku* (forest bathing), given all the beautifully landscaped gardens and tree-lined streets in my neighborhood. It was the same for my husband, who also incorporated more cycling into the mix.

We saved money. We were gentler to the earth. The planning got easier. But the biggest benefit was the sense of community we developed. Because we needed rides everywhere, we formed stronger bonds with neighbors and friends. We simply saw them more, impromptu get-togethers emerging from carpooling. Eventually we bought another car, but the lessons I learned during that six-month carless phase have stuck with me. Life felt simpler and lovelier.

Now, in the second half of my life, I find myself intentionally seeking that shibui simplicity. I still opt out of driving whenever possible and walk for miles every day. I reach out and arrange coffee dates with friends. I slow down and weigh the value of each activity. My time without a car felt beautifully shibui, and I've carried that quieter, simpler, somehow more essentially connected feeling into my current days.

Aging with grace means that sometimes, what appears to be a limitation can enhance our lives, creating space for the connections and experiences that truly matter. Like a carefully pruned bonsai tree, constraints can shape us into something more beautiful and meaningful than unlimited growth ever could.

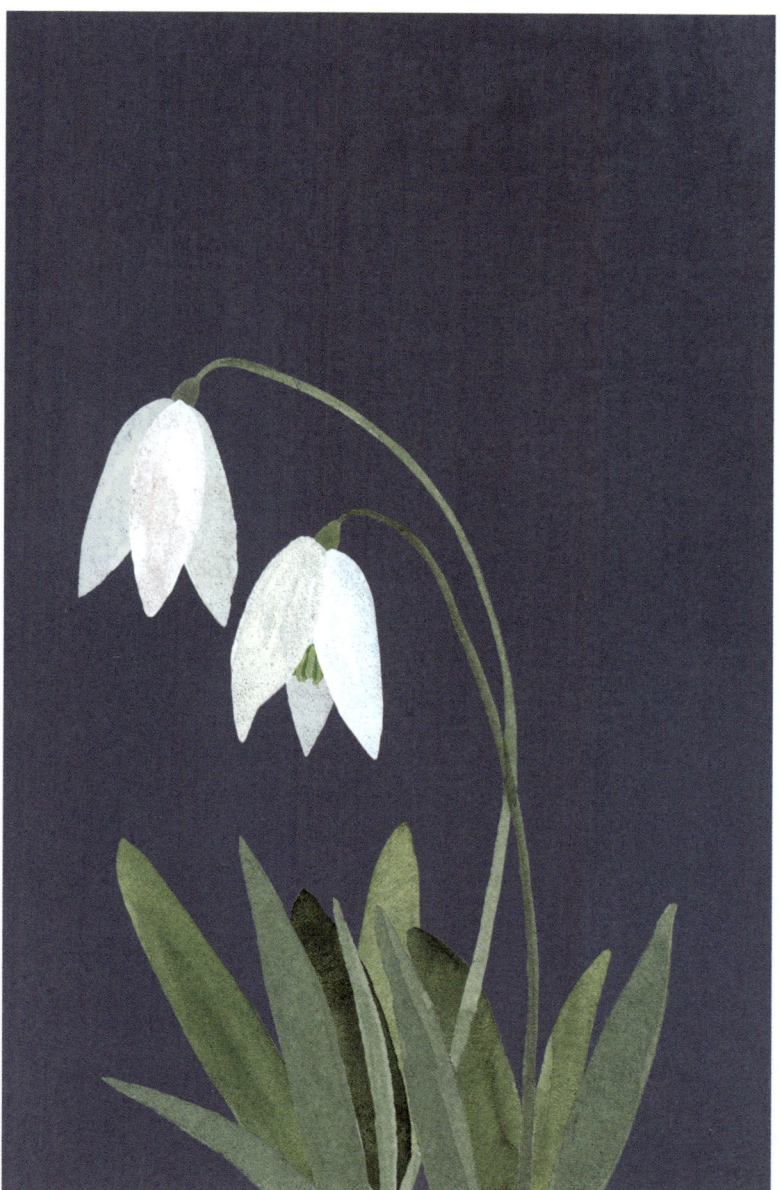

In the end, only three things matter:
How much you loved,
How gently you lived,
And how gracefully you let go
of the things not meant for you.

COMMONLY ATTRIBUTED TO BUDDHA

終わり

Owari

THE ENDING

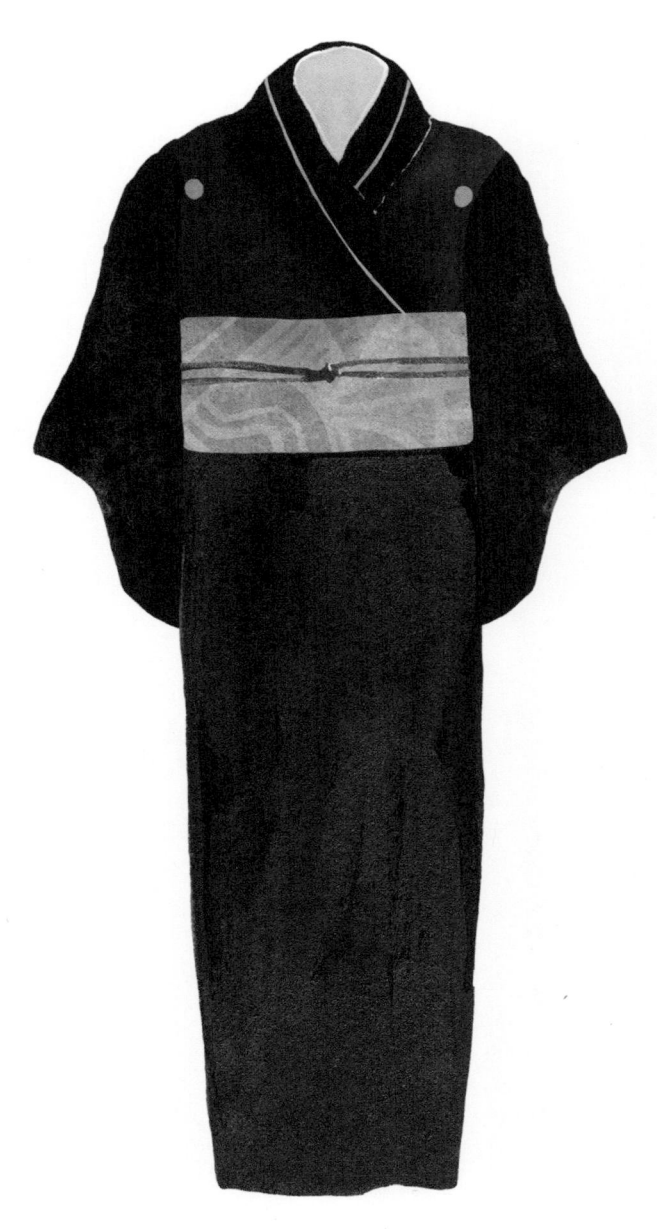

ON DYING

WE ARE ALL GOING to die. You, me, everyone. As a Japanese-American woman, I've surmised that the sharpest delineation between the two cultures is in their attitudes toward death. Americans treat death like a rumor that appears to be based on truth but one that no one believes. The rumor is whispered behind closed doors, eyes sliding away in discomfort. The Japanese have no compunction about discussing the end of life. I grew up listening to my parents discuss death in the same breath as coordinating my brother's Little League games.

True shibui embraces the full spectrum of life, including its finitude. The beauty is in accepting the natural rhythm of existence, including the inevitability of endings.

Owari can be both "the ending" and "the end." A singular owari graces many a Japanese picture book. Death, too, is like the end of a story filled with words and images. And if we're lucky, we will have lived a shibui tale to be told.

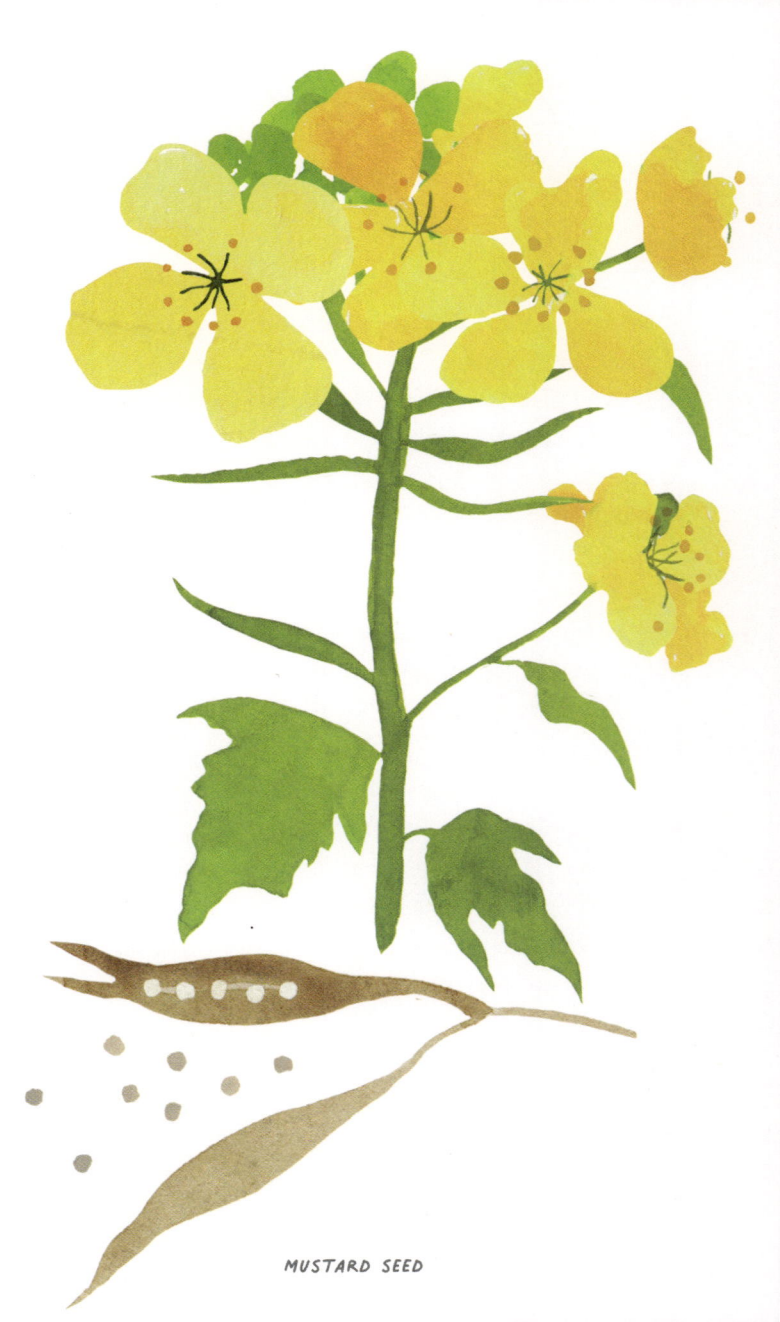

MUSTARD SEED

THE WHITE MUSTARD SEED

THERE IS A WELL-KNOWN Buddhist parable that gains more significance as I age. It concerns Kisa Gotami, whose son has died. Denying his death, she believes he is merely asleep and visits one house after another, seeking medicine to wake him. Eventually Buddha offers to help if she brings him a white mustard seed from a family untouched by death.

Kisa Gotami knocks on door after door but cannot find a single family that hasn't experienced death. She returns to Buddha empty-handed, understanding that pain, suffering, and death are unavoidable parts of life. Thus enlightened, she becomes a nun.

Now I'm happy to skip the nun ordination, but the lesson is valuable. John Muth adapted this story into a picture book, replacing the mustard seed with a sugar bowl. Bittersweet, just like shibui.

This fable reminds us of the universality of loss. Rather than seeing death as something to fear or deny, it acknowledges death as the natural conclusion to life's story. There is a quiet elegance in this acceptance—not resignation, but a clear-eyed understanding that makes our limited time more precious.

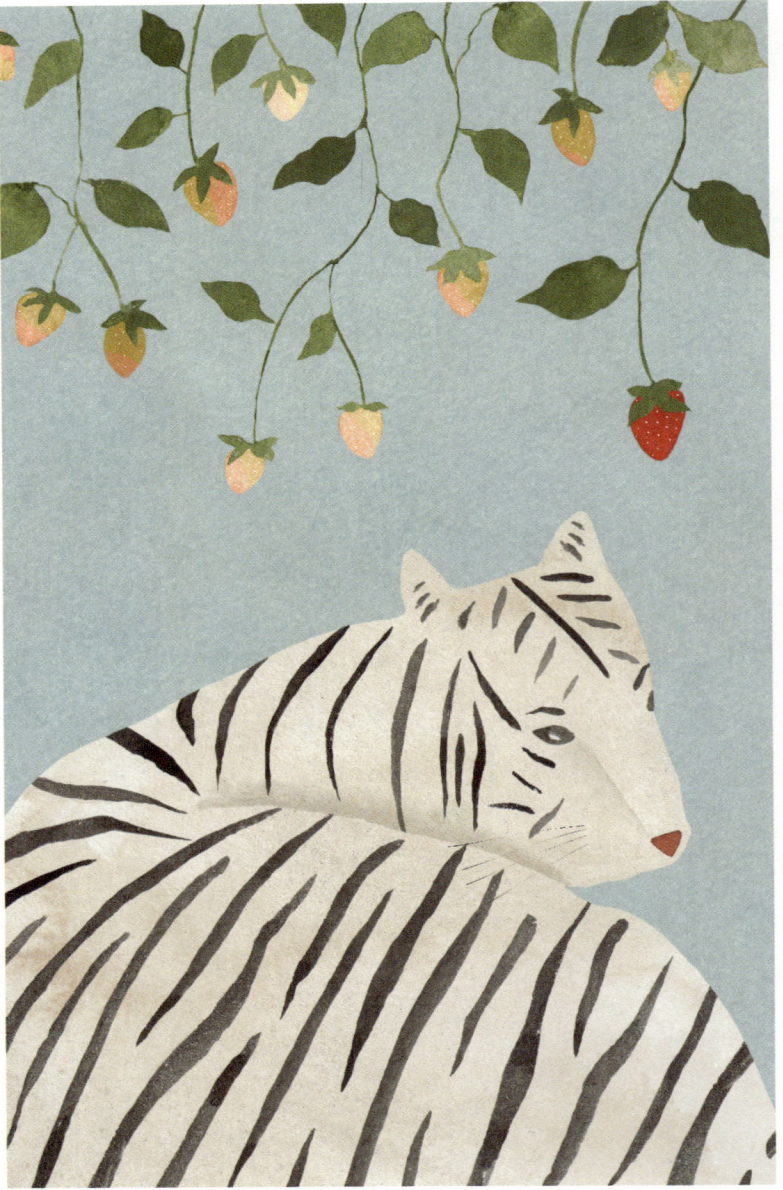

ICHIGO ICHIE (AND A STORY ABOUT TIGERS AND STRAWBERRIES)

ANOTHER FAVORITE PARABLE NOT only discusses death but also the choices we make while we live:

> One day a man turns to find that a ferocious tiger is chasing him. The man runs with all his might, but he keeps checking over his shoulder and doesn't see the cliff ahead. He runs right off the edge, Wile E. Coyote style, and falls straight down. Instinctively the man shoots out his arm and grasps a branch that breaks his fall a short way from the ground. He looks up, only to see the tiger growling hungrily, its spittle flying about. He looks down and sees the darkest void. Above: death by tiger. Below: death by fall. An untenable situation. Then the man notices a single brilliantly red and perfectly ripe strawberry right by the branch he grips. He plucks the strawberry and pops it in his mouth, closing his eyes and savoring the juicy sweetness.

This little story aptly captures the Japanese idiom *ichigo ichie*, which is essentially about treasuring the unrepeatable nature of the present moment. Just as we can never cross the river at the exact same spot, no two moments are ever exactly alike. Death is a guarantee, and life is all the sweeter for it. Although "ichigo" in the idiom translates to one's lifetime in Buddhist terms, it also means "strawberry" in Japanese (spelled differently, however). Ichigo ichie, in its fullest definition, is the uniqueness of each experience: one encounter, one lifetime.

As we age, living in a shibui way invites us to become more attentive to these fleeting, singular moments—to notice and relish the metaphorical strawberries in our daily lives. The awareness of our mortality can sharpen our joy rather than diminish it. Like the man holding onto the branch, we find ourselves suspended between the past and the future, with only the present moment truly in our grasp.

Obon Celebration

Every year in mid-August, millions of Japanese people descend upon seaside towns or attend local festivals to celebrate Obon, a three-day Japanese festival in honor of the deceased, a celebration that is similar to the Western All Souls' Day or Mexico's Day of the Dead. Obon pays tribute to, the deceased and welcomes back, the ancestral spirits from the land of the dead.

During Obon, fireworks light up the nighttime skies, and street vendors hawk skewers of grilled chicken, noodle dishes, taiyaki (fish-shaped pastries filled with red bean paste), takoyaki (a savory ball-shaped cooked wheat dough filled with chopped octopus), and many other delectable fares.

Folks dress up in summer kimonos, dance to taiko beats, and play traditional games such as scooping up goldfish. Obon is one of the most important events in Japan. Like the shibui understanding that life is transient, Obon is an enthusiastic nod to the impermanent cycle of life and views it as celebratory.

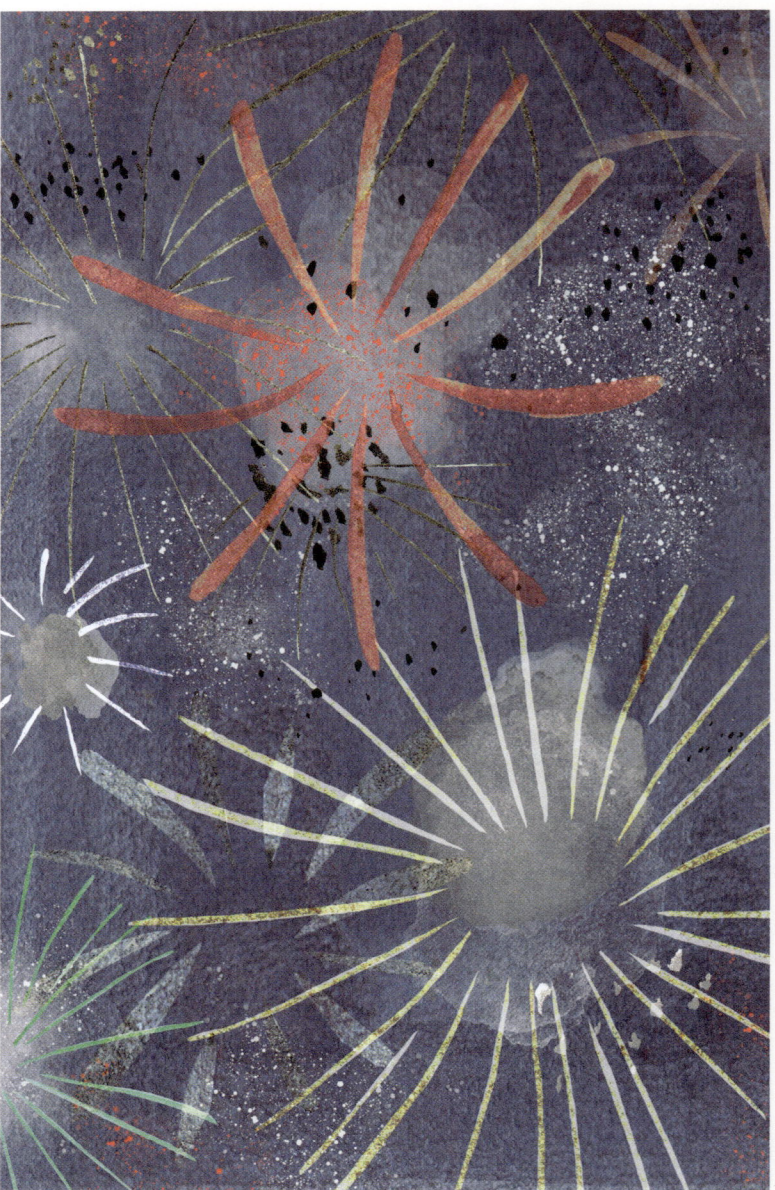

THE AFTERMATH (AFTERLIFE)
AND QUIRMING

DEATH AND DECAY ARE very much a part of the shibui mentality. Nothing on earth lasts, but there is beauty in the ephemeral. Did you know that ephemeral plants wait out droughts as seeds? I like to think of death as a period of drought, a cycle of fallowness. The essence of me remains and will reemerge when it's time to flourish, perhaps as a different being.

The perspective that a temporarily housed soul spirits to a different mortal home once a life cycle completes brings a certain lightness to aging—each wrinkle and gray hair not a step toward an end but a mark of progress in a much longer journey.

Lately I've been reading many Japanese books translated into English. Often infused with magical surrealism, they have a quirky, charming quality I call "*quirming.*" They feature restaurants that "investigate" nostalgic dishes, libraries filled with only books to ease sorrows, or time-traveling cafés. Deceased characters and ghosts appear prominently, portrayed with an almost lighthearted quality.

Yes, the Japanese make death quirming, something to be wholly accepted and even appreciated—something that perhaps we shouldn't take too seriously.

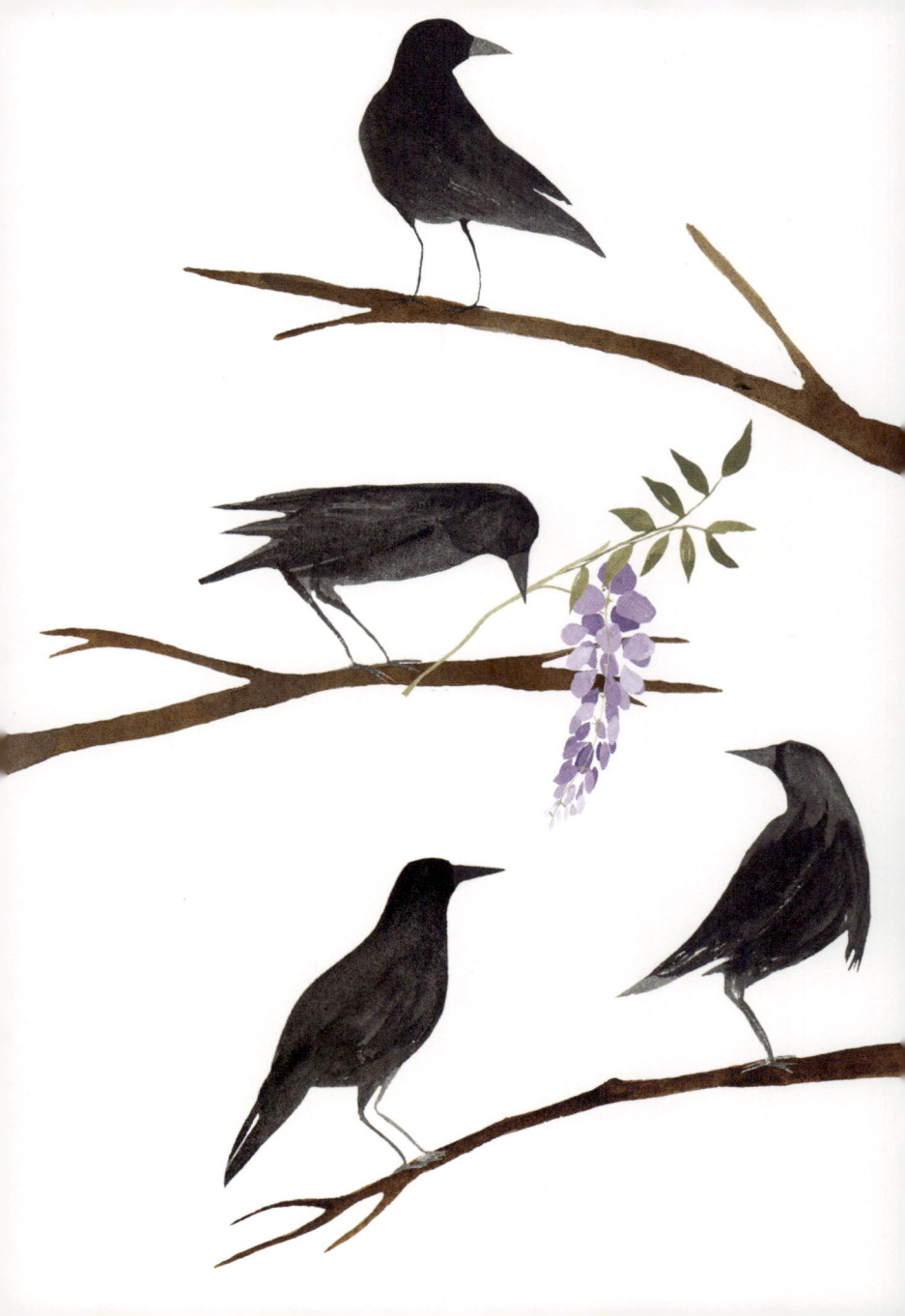

THE CROWS

A FEW SUMMERS AGO, I was walking up a hill when, with a *swoosh,* something heavy and smooth brushed against my head. Startled, I stopped to see what it was. A crow landed several feet from me and stared. Its wing had caressed my hair! We studied each other for several beats, then I resumed moving. Then just a couple of days later, while I was walking down an entirely different street in a different neighborhood, another crow tapped me on my shoulder. The touch was gentle, decidedly friendly.

Incredibly, days later more crows showed up. Again I was in a neighboring area, separate from the other two occasions, when I noticed that a crow was hopping alongside me. On the other side, another crow began hopping to match the first. Hop, swoop, hop. The two crows accompanied me for two blocks, and then, through some silent signal, both birds simultaneously flew away. I was getting spooked.

The following week, my daughter and I were chatting in the kitchen, which sits at the back of the house. To cool our unairconditioned home, we'd left the front door open with the screen door shut. Due to an incident with our toddler neighbor, the lower portion of the screen door had been knocked out. My daughter and I heard a scuffling noise, and as I approached the front of the house, I saw that a crow was trying to enter through the gap! Frightened, I immediately shut the door.

Finally, upon returning from a morning walk, I spotted *four* crows in front of the house. They watched me open the door with my key, then flew off. "They've been waiting for you," my daughter joked. I think she may have been right.

The crows left me alone after that.

In Japan crows are one of the holiest birds, akin to herons. They signify wisdom and guidance—qualities associated with aging. They are also heralds of disturbance and death. Ultimately the crow—intelligent, adaptable, and often misunderstood—embodies certain aspects of shibui aging. They are neither purely beautiful nor purely ominous but complex creatures that defy simple categorization. Initially I'd worried about impending demise but then opted to interpret this eerie yet magical few weeks as a sign of heightened guidance: to cherish my life and to age well.

Japanese Symbols of Death

Nuanced symbolisms of death reflect the shibui philosophy—finding beauty and meaning in life's inevitable conclusion. These symbols remind us that aging and mortality are natural parts of existence, to be acknowledged rather than denied.

BUTTERFLY: This insect represents both the soul of the deceased and transformation. Butterflies are also associated with menopause, symbolizing the transition to a new stage of life.

SHI (DEATH, THE NUMBER FOUR): The kanji characters for "death" and "four" differ, but their similar pronunciation (shi) makes the number four symbolic of death in Japanese culture, and it is typically interpreted as unlucky. Just as Western buildings often omit the thirteenth floor, Japanese elevators might skip the fourth floor or floors forty to forty-nine.

RED SPIDER LILY: These striking red flowers bloom around the autumnal equinox, coinciding with Ohigan, a Buddhist holiday for remembering ancestors. Frequently planted around cemeteries, their appearance signals the transition between worlds.

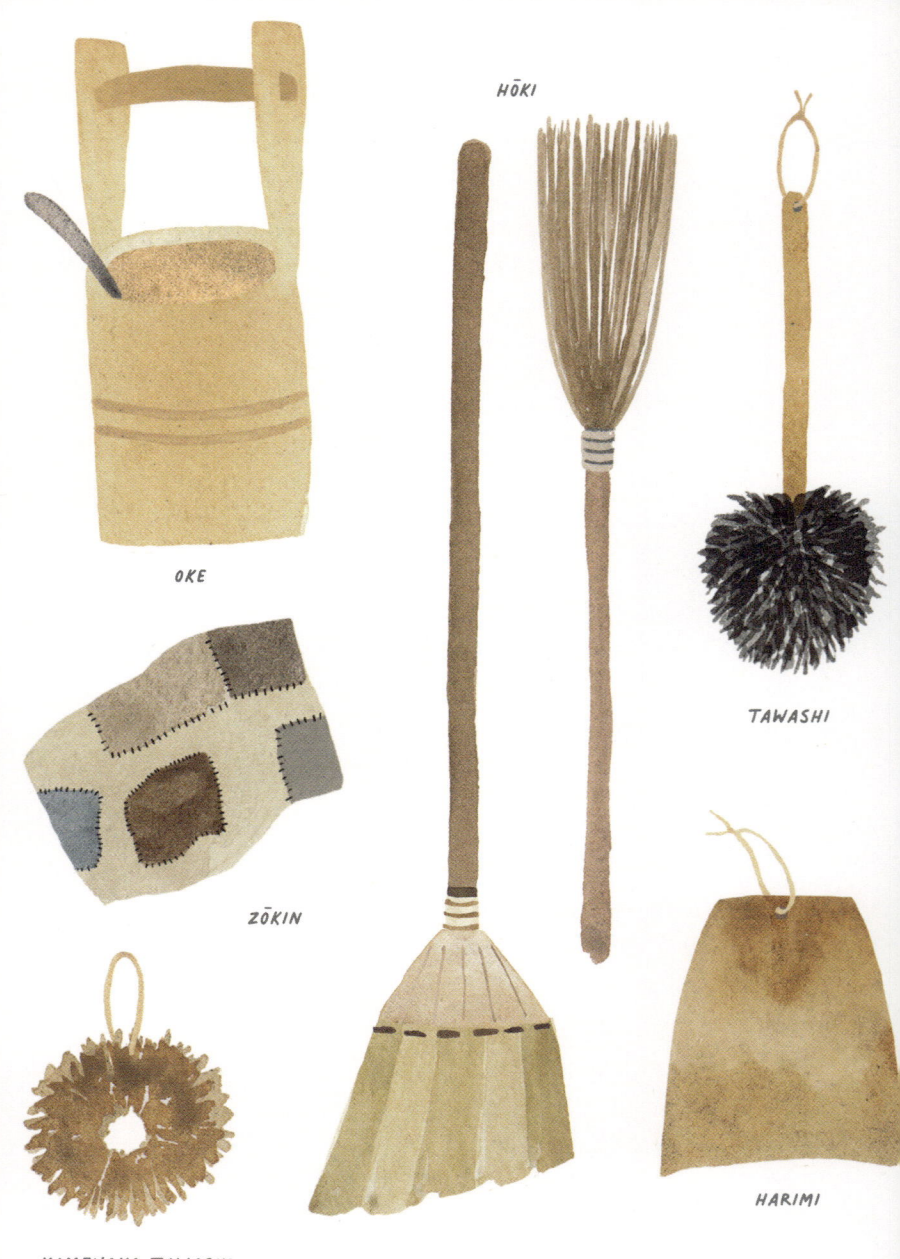

HŌKI

OKE

TAWASHI

ZŌKIN

KAMENOKO TAWASHI

HARIMI

KIREIZUKI

MY MOM IS A maximalist. She fills every surface and space with stuff. Growing up, to make my way through the house I had to jump over her art canvases and shove aside her collections of Godzilla toys, vintage signage, and a mountain of craft supplies. This tendency toward maximalism (let's be honest, hoarding) stems from an upbringing that she describes as *binbō* (poor).

Japanese homes exhibit fascinating extremes. There are the ingrained cultural values of minimalism and visual expansiveness—essential in a small country with limited space. Yet many Japanese homes I visited were packed with tchotchkes and would qualify to be featured on the television show, *Hoarders*. My childhood home would have been too, and with every video call I've caught glimpses of my parents' stockpiling clutter at a dizzying clip in their new home in Japan.

Maybe it's a reaction to my childhood, but I maintain more of a minimalist environment in my own little townhouse. During visits, my mother calls me *kireizuki*—someone with a penchant for cleanliness and an appreciation for lovely things. I'll take it.

The Swedish death cleaning concept encourages decluttering while alive to spare family members from dealing with the household remains later. Knowing the enormous task awaiting me when my mom passes, I've adopted this mentality toward my own material possessions. I'm eager to unburden myself in the here and now as much as possible (shimmery taupe eyeshadow notwithstanding) to lighten the load for my daughter or any other surviving family members as I prepare for my eventual "reincarnation expedition." I'm proud to be kireizuki.

Pre-Death Cleaning Ritual

How do you feel about Swedish death cleaning? What will you leave behind?

Here are the few space-efficient items I plan to keep:

- Favorite photos (mostly digitized)
- My daughter's childhood memorabilia, such as the small sculptures of her hand and foot made by my father-in-law
- Select artwork by my mom, myself, and a few treasured artists
- My most cherished books, but not too many

With a move on the near horizon, I'm further motivated to downsize and evaluate what's truly worth keeping. I need so little, and I find it freeing to release my grip on things—a beautifully shibui approach to creating inner and outer spaciousness.

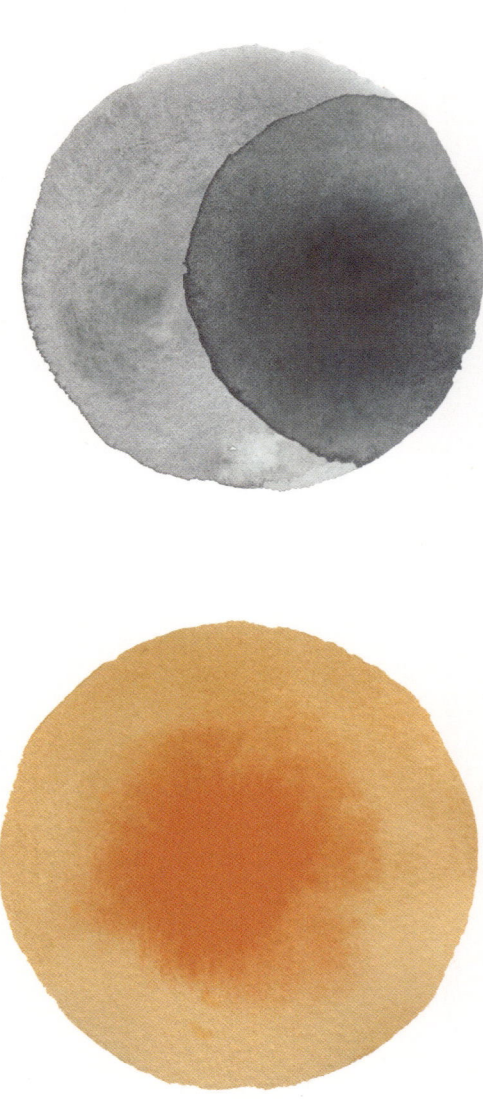

CONCLUSION

MY DAUGHTER LEFT FOR college recently, and as I was cleaning and organizing our house in full empty-nesting mode, I came across one of her elementary school assignments. She was tasked with creating an acrostic: a poem in which she ascribes a descriptor for each letter of her name. Inspired, I considered one for shibui:

S = simple
H = harmonious
I = imperfect
B = beautiful
U = unpretentious
I = impermanent

My acrostic dovetails nicely with the seven qualities commonly attributed to shibui, which are simplicity, implicitness, modesty, silence, naturalness, everydayness, and imperfection.

Shibui is not easily defined and can be likened to a river. The ebb and flow of the currents feel like the vicissitudes of active and immersed living, but there is a profound stillness that reigns within and beneath. In many ways, the reflection of the water forms a moving mirror of our inner world.

A river is perfectly imperfect—for have you ever seen one that's symmetrical like a highway? In its imperfection, it is harmonious with all of nature. It is, quite literally, down-to-earth. In the ichigo ichie spirit, you cannot step into the same part of the river twice, and like everything else on this mysterious planet of ours, it is impermanent. Apparently as rivers age, they become wider, not deeper. The metaphor still holds for me. As we age, we gain not merely depth but breadth. A more hiroi presence, if you will. If we allow it, we develop an abiding ability to forgive ourselves and others for our humanity, to find worth in our simple existence, to undo the disease of loneliness, and find solace in quiet solitude while remaining intertwined with all sentient beings. We become an expanse of experience, wisdom, and openness.

I invite you to wholeheartedly dive into your own shibui flow to discover the unique beauty that emerges as you age. May you find, as I have, that though the passing years will not prevent flaws, limitations, and loss, they serve to enrich, transform, and unveil life's most precious gifts. Let us love heartily, live gently, and release gracefully all that's not meant for us—let's savor all the mellowed sweetness of aging.

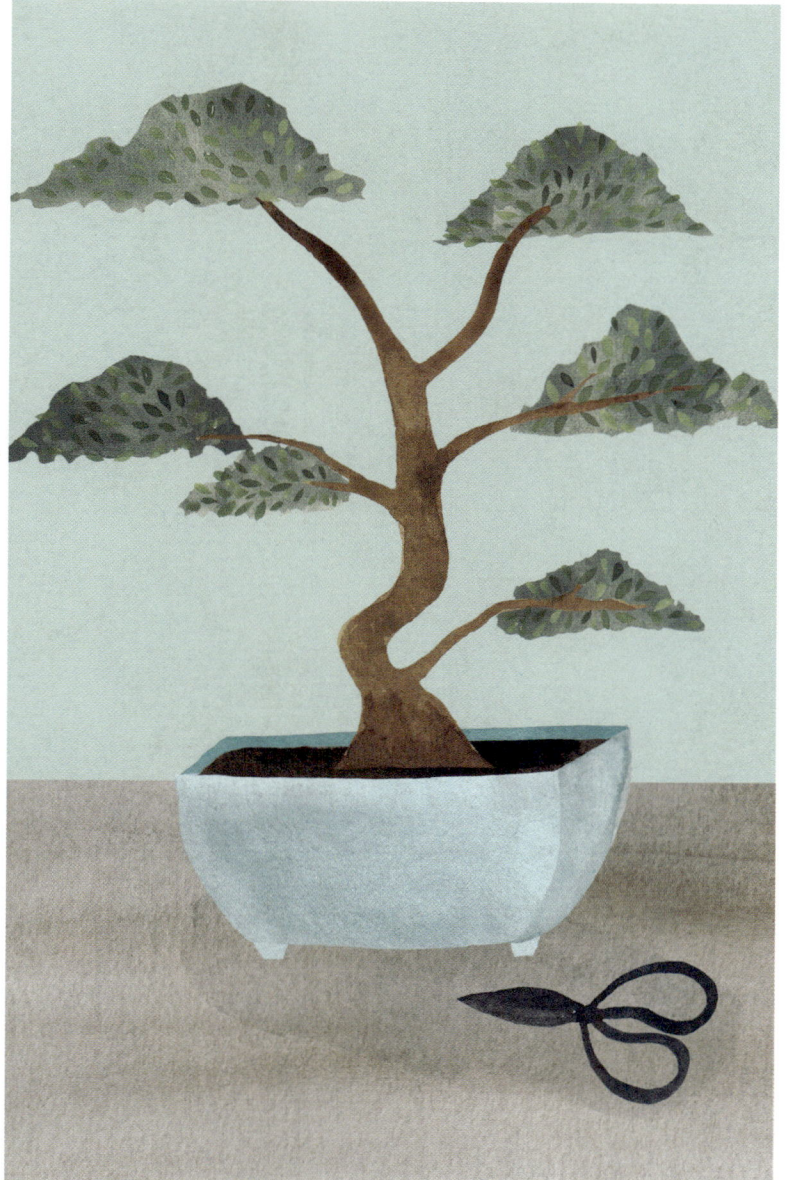

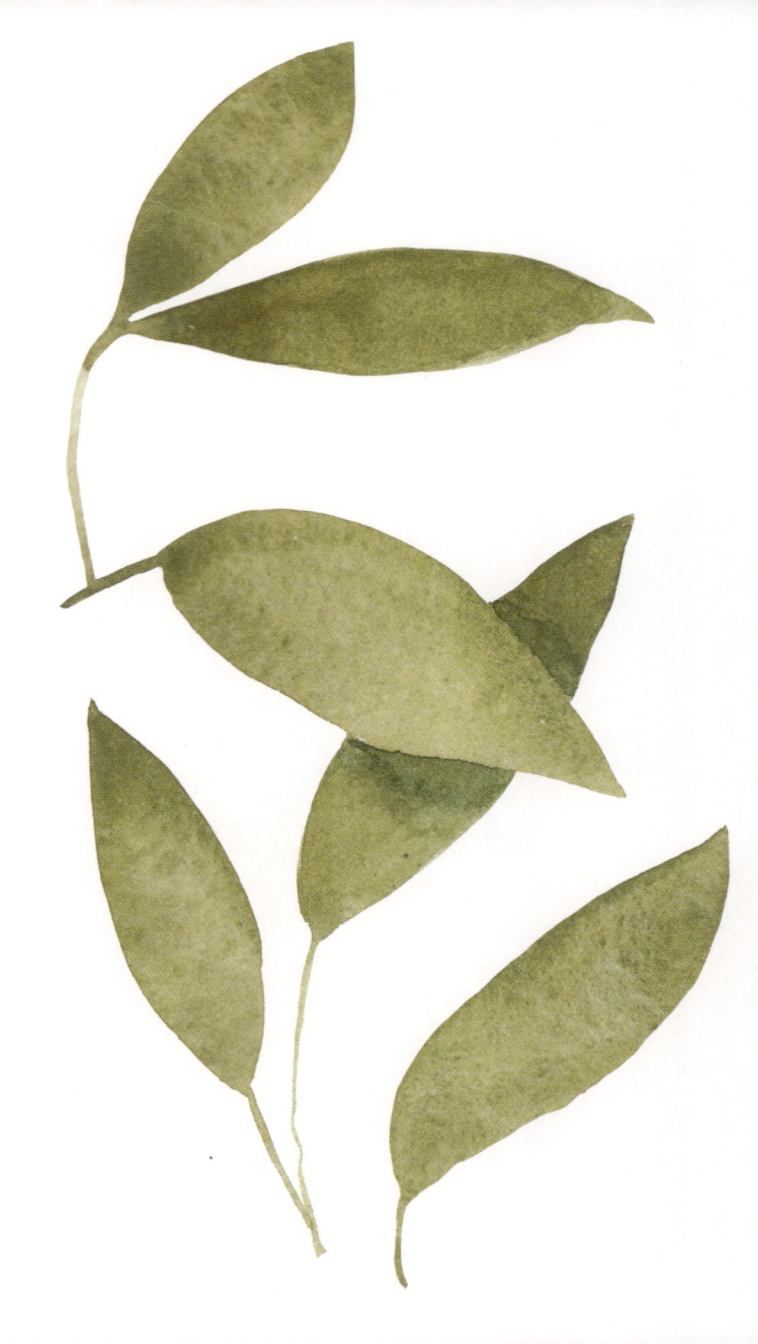

GLOSSARY OF JAPANESE TERMS

AI (愛): Love; a deep, committed form of love

BANCHA (番茶): Green tea made from the second harvest of the same plant as sencha, but with larger leaves

BINBŌ (貧乏): Poor or impoverished

BONSAI (盆栽): Meticulously pruned miniature trees

BORO (ぼろ / つぎはぎ): The practice of mending and patching textiles; boro means "tattered" or "repaired," and tsugihagi refers to patchwork of scraps

CHA (茶): Tea

CHIE (智慧): Wisdom

CHIRI MO TSUMOREBA, YAMA TO NARU (塵も積もれば 山となる): "Even small particles of dust, when accumulated, can become a mountain"; proverb about the power of small, consistent actions

DAISUKI (大好き): "Big like"; a stronger form of affection than suki, often translated as "love"

EIYŌ (栄養): Nourishment; holistic sustenance that goes beyond mere nutrition

FŪRIN (風鈴): Japanese word for wind chime

GENKI (元気): Energetic, lively, full of vitality; "gen" means origin/source, and "ki" refers to life force

GENMAICHA (玄米茶): Sencha plus roasted rice. Nutty with sesame-like flavor. Less caffeine

GOCHISŌSAMA (ごちそうさま): "Thank you for the meal" or "It was a feast"; said after finishing a meal

GOYA (ごや): Bitter melon or bitter gourd; a staple produce in Okinawa

HARA HACHI BU (腹八分): Eating until you are 80 percent full; a principle of moderation. HARAHACHIBUNME (腹八分目) means the same thing

HARIMI (はりみ): Traditional Japanese dustpan made of thick paper layers cured with persimmon tannin

HIGANBANA (彼岸花): Spider lily or magic lily; a flower associated with death and the afterlife

HIROI (広い): Spacious, expansive; often used to describe one's heart or mind (kokoro)

HŌJICHA (ほうじ茶 or 焙じ茶): Roasted green tea leaves. Very little caffeine with a rich, earthy taste

HŌKI (ほうき): Japanese word for broom

HOSHIGAKI (干し柿): Dried persimmons

ICHIGO (いちご): Strawberry

ICHIGO ICHIE (一期一会): "One moment, one encounter"; a concept emphasizing the uniqueness and transience of each moment

IKIGAI (生きがい): A reason for being; purpose in life

IREZUMI (入れ墨): Japanese word for tattoo, often associated with yakuza

ITADAKIMASU (いただきます): "I humbly receive"; said before eating a meal

KAKI (柿): Persimmon

KAME (亀): Turtle

KAMENOKO TAWASHI (亀の子たわし): Circular scrubbing brush

KAMPŌ (漢方): Japanese traditional medicine adapted from Chinese methodologies

KANSHA (感謝): Gratitude, thanksgiving

KARŌSHI (過労死): Death from overwork

KENKŌ (健康): Health or healthy

KENSHŌ (見性): First insight or initial awakening in Zen Buddhism

KI (気): Life force or energy that flows through all living things

KIMONO (着物): Traditional Japanese garment worn by men and women

KINTSUGI (金継ぎ): The art of repairing broken pottery with gold-infused lacquer

KITSUNE (狐 or きつね): Fox

KIREIZUKI (綺麗好き): Someone with a penchant for cleanliness and an appreciation for lovely things

KOKORO (心): Heart/mind; refers to both the emotional and intellectual aspects of being

KŌNENKI (更年期): Menopause; a time of renewal in Japanese culture

KOTSU-KOTSU (コツコツ): Working diligently in small measures

MANEKI-NEKO (招き猫): A beckoning cat associated with prosperity; small ceramic figurines placed at the entrance of shops to invite abundance

MATCHA (抹茶): Powdered tencha leaves. Bright green and has more caffeine

MIEPPARI (見栄っ張り): A person overly concerned with appearances or status

MIKAN (みかん): Mandarin oranges

MINGEI (民芸): Folk art movement founded by Dr. Soetsu Yanagi

MIZUHIKI KNOTS(水引): Traditionally formed out of thin washi paper strips to adorn gifts. Used as celebratory decoration

MOAI (模合): Traditional social support groups in Okinawa

MOCHI (もち): Japanese rice cake made from glutinous rice pounded into a sticky dough; plays a prominent role in New Year celebrations

MOKUTEKI (目的): Purpose, objective

MOMO (桃): Peach, peach tree

NADESHIKO (撫子): Dianthus superbus; flower associated with feminine beauty

OBON (お盆): Annual festival honoring ancestral spirits

OHIGAN (お彼岸): Buddhist holiday for remembering ancestors

OKASĀN (お母さん): Mother

OKE (桶): Japanese wooden bucket typically made of hinoki used for bathing

OSOZAKI (遅咲き): Late or slow blooms; late bloomers

ŌBAI TŌRI (桜梅桃李): Concept referring to the unique beauty of different flowering trees, symbolizing the importance of acknowledging individual strengths and avoiding comparison

OWARI (終わり or 終り): The ending; the end

RADIO TAISO (ラジオ体操): Radio calisthenics; morning exercises performed at schools and workplaces

RI (李): Apricot, apricot tree

SABI (寂): A beauty that comes with age; patina

SALARIMAN (サラリーマン): Salaried worker, typically in a corporate environment

SAKURA (桜): Cherry blossom or cherry tree

SASHIKO (刺し子): A form of decorative and/or reinforcement stitching

SEMAI (狭い): Narrow, constricted

SENCHA (煎茶): Green tea made from the first harvest. Very mild with a little bit of caffeine

SHI (死/四): Death/the number four; considered unlucky due to similar pronunciation

SHIBUI (渋い): Having an understated, subtle, and unobtrusive beauty that emerges with time

SHIBUMI/SHIBUSA (渋み/渋さ): The noun form of shibui; the astringent taste of an unripe persimmon; bitterness

SHIGOTO (仕事): Work, job, occupation

SHINRINYOKU (森林浴): Forest bathing; spending time in forests for wellbeing

SHINTŌ (神道): A religious practice in Japan that means "the way of the god" or "the way of gods"

SHISA (シーサー): Lion-dog or lion-dragon statues in Okinawan culture that serve as guardians

SHISO (紫蘇): Perilla; a herb used in Japanese cooking

SHOGI (将棋): A strategy game played by two people, similar to chess

SHUYAKU (主役): Main character or starring role

SŌSAKU (創作): Creativity or creative work

SUKI (好き): Like or love; a lighter form of affection

TAIKO (太鼓): Japanese drum

TAKOYAKI (たこ焼き or 蛸焼): A savory ball-shaped cooked wheat dough filled with chopped octopus

TAKUAN (沢庵): Pickled daikon radish

TAIYAKI (鯛焼き): Fish-shaped pastries filled with red bean paste

TANTANTO (淡々と): Going with the flow in a light, detached manner

TANUKI (狸, たぬき): Racoon dog

TAWASHI (たわし): Scrubbing brush

TENCHA (碾茶): The purest form of green tea leaves without veins, stems, stalks, etc.

TOMI (富): Wealth, abundance

TSUGIHAGI (継ぎ接ぎ): Patchwork

TSUNAGARI (繋がり): Connection, relationship, bond

URAYAMASHII (羨ましい): A positive form of envy or admiration without bitterness

URUSHI (漆): *Toxicodendron vernicifluum*, also known as the Chinese lacquer tree. In traditional kintsugi, the sap is used as the decorative laquer and glue to hold broken pottery pieces together

UME (梅): Plum, plum blossom or plum tree

WABI (侘): Imperfection; harmonious beauty

WAKI-YAKU (脇役): Supporting role or character

YAKUZA (ヤクザ): Organized crime groups in Japan; Japanese mafia

YAMAI WA KI KARA (病は気から): "Sickness and health start with the mind"; Japanese proverb

YUTAKA (豊か): Rich, abundant, prosperous; describes a life of leisurely abundance

YUTORI (ゆとり): Spaciousness, room to breathe; mental and physical space that allows for relaxation and creativity

ZŌKIN (雑巾): Cleaning cloth

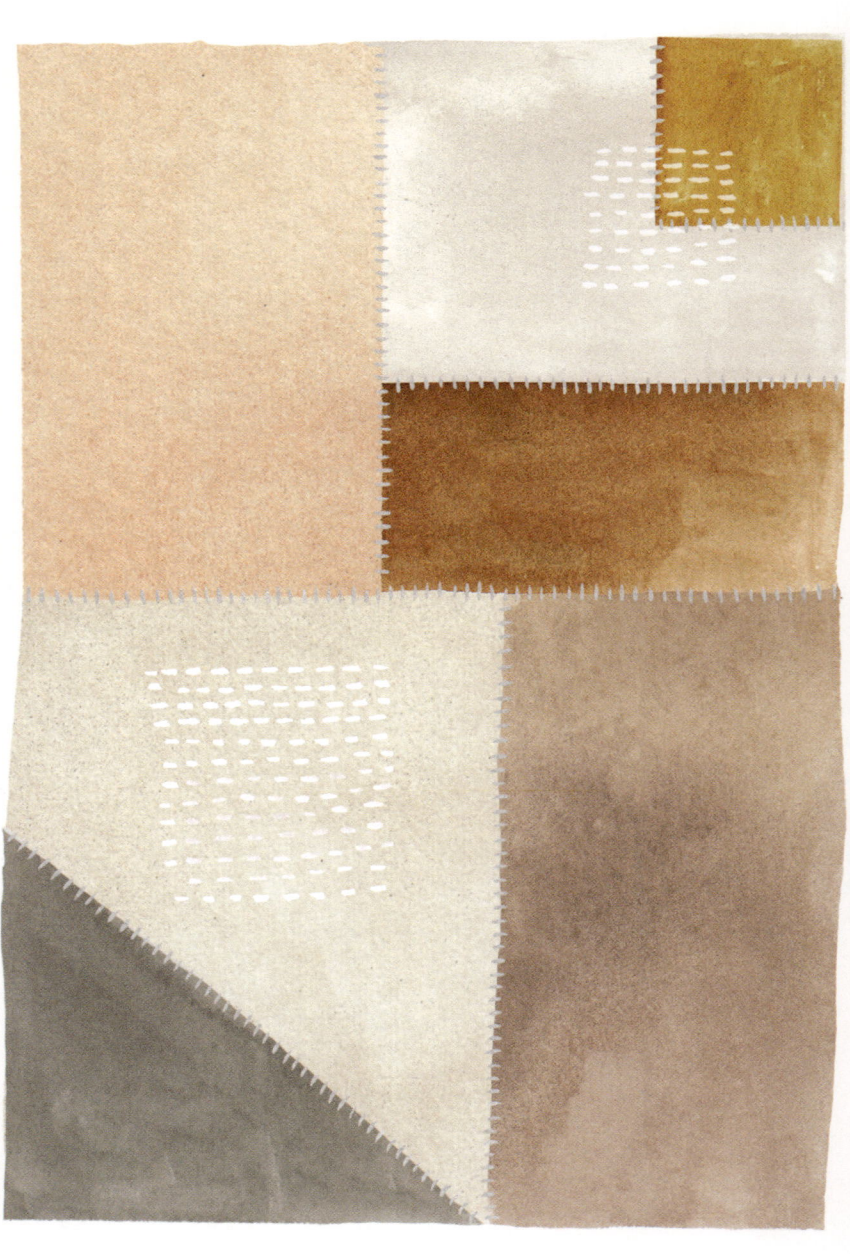

ACKNOWLEDGMENTS

IMMEASURABLE KANSHA FOR THE many people involved with this little book with a lot of heart. First and foremost, editor extraordinaire and wonderful friend Hannah Elnan: a few years ago, you said to me, "That idea you had about aging—there's something juicy there." *Shibui* is dedicated to you. With Anna Goldstein (art director extraordinaire!), we sculpted the proposal, and it's hard to believe that it is now an actual, real book. To Avalon Radys, thank you for making the transition a smooth and lovely one! Great big thanks to *all* the amazing folks at Sasquatch Books past and present—I'm blown away by the care and magnitude of effort required for each book.

A special shout-out to the picture book support group, whose enthusiastic encouragement spurred me on. To Adria Goetz, thank you for being an intrepid and kind agent. Much thanks to my fortifying and generous Furoku/Patreon members. Dearest readers and knowledgeable booksellers, *arigatou* (thank you).

And to my beautiful, stalwart family and friends who are consistently very confused about what I actually do (as am I), I love you more than words can express. I feel lucky that I'm growing older with you all.

Printed in China

SASQUATCH BOOKS with colophon is a registered
trademark of Blue Star Press, LLC

29 28 27 26 25   9 8 7 6 5 4 3 2

EU Rep: Authorised Rep Compliance Ltd., Ground Floor,
71 Lower Baggot Street, Dublin, D02 P593, Ireland.
www.arccompliance.com.

Editor: Avalon Radys
Production editor: Peggy Gannon
Designer: Anna Goldstein

Library of Congress Cataloging-in-Publication Data is available

ISBN: 978-1-63217-575-5

Sasquatch Books
1325 Fourth Avenue, Suite 1025
Seattle, WA 98101

SasquatchBooks.com